# Life Change

Barbara Evans qualified in medicine from the Royal Free Hospital in London. After training as a pathologist she investigated anaemia in pregnant women in Bombay, ran an emergency laboratory in England during the war, and worked in the United States and Vietnam. *Caduceus in Saigon* was published in 1968. She was the medical correspondent of the *Sunday Times* for several years and is now Managing Editor of *World Medicine*. Having married soon after graduation, she has also had a full family life with three sons, one daughter, and eight grandchildren, so far.

Dr Barbara Evans

# Life Change

A Guide to the Menopause, its Effects
and Treatment

with a foreword by Mr John Studd MD MRCOG

Pan Original
Pan Books London and Sydney

Acknowledgement: I'd like to thank the women who told me their stories, and the gynaecologists who let me visit their menopause clinics: Mr Robert Beard, Professor Stuart Campbell, Mr Michael Pugh and Mr John Studd. I'm especially grateful to Mr Studd for writing the foreword and for his enthusiasm and help, and to Dr Anne Anderson who stopped me from sticking my neck out too far; also to Mr Elliot Philipp, the late Dr J. M. Slattery and Professor A. C. Turnbull for advice. The busiest people always help you most and are the most fun to work with.

First published 1979 by Pan Books Ltd,
Cavaye Place, London SW10 9PG,
in association with William Collins & Co Ltd
3rd printing 1979
© Barbara Evans 1979
ISBN 0 330 25628 9
Printed and bound in Great Britain by
Hazell Watson & Viney Ltd, Aylesbury, Bucks

for my last good egg

Like the first appearance, so the cessation of the periods varies in different subjects, and is in subordination to the temperament, the constitution, the climate and the habit of life of the female.

*Colombat de L'Isière, 1845. Resident Surgeon of the Maison de Santé, of the Rue de Valois du Roule.*

Some diseases at the change of life escape all explanation.

*E. J. Tilt, 1851. Senior Physician to the Farringdon General Dispensary and Lying-in Charity, and to the Paddington Free Dispensary for the Diseases of Women and Children.*

# Contents

# Foreword

Dr Barbara Evans' scholarly account of the menopause appears in press at an opportune time as the question of hormone replacement therapy is at the crossroads of a major medical controversy. Oestrogen therapy is not a panacea for all ills, nor does it contain a rejuvenation promise of 'feminine forever', but it does remove unpleasant physical and psychological symptoms of oestrogen deficiency in the middle-aged. It is appropriate that, as the benefits are well documented and beyond dispute, investigators are now studying the potential side effects of thrombosis, diabetes and, above all, cancer of the lining of the womb. As British women are demanding oestrogen therapy, their American sisters are becoming reluctant to take the implied risk. The Food and Drugs Administration has instructed that a warning health hazard notice be included in packets of oestrogens, and American gynaecologists wait in dread anticipation for litigation claims. Such is the dilemma of a therapy which on one hand promised so much in the area of preventive medicine, but has invoked fearful alarms of lethal complications.

The years after the menopause should be regarded as a hormone-deficient state, in the same way as diabetes. The hormone insulin is usually required for the treatment of diabetes and the fact that insulin has side effects and such therapy may not correct all the many hazards of the disease in no way alters the truth of this definition.

British research into the menopause is now focused on these side effects in order to determine the correct selection of patients and the correct dose of a natural or synthetic oestrogen. We must also determine if there is a cancer risk, and if so, what balance of hormones must be used to avoid overstimulation of the lining of the womb.

This book captures the excitement of this most important

area of medicine and I have no doubt that the reader will find the text fascinating and, above all, will finish this well-researched account of the menopause better informed than many who allow women to sweat out their distress in a haze of emotional debility and tranquillizers.

John Studd MD MRCOG, King's College Hospital, London

# Preface

Some societies reward women for their services to the race when they reach the end of their fertility, giving them the freedom and often the status which they had lacked during their reproductive years. Women from countries where age is venerated suffer less physically than other women at the change of life, or menopause. Unfortunately, ours is not one of those societies.

The life expectancy of women has increased from 45 to 70 years during this century. But although women now live longer, unfortunately their ovaries do not. These begin to fail on average between 45 and 52 years of age, leaving women to spend approximately a third of their lives after the decline in ovarian function. There are four to five million women in the United Kingdom at this stage now. Of those women who suffer from resulting menopausal distress, which can be very severe in a minority, a large number are still denied treatment. This is particularly regrettable since the results of treatment when properly applied can be remarkable. Once the problem is recognized, most, if not all, the troubles of the menopause can usually be alleviated, and need no longer be regarded as inevitable. Many British women and some doctors still do not appear to realize that help is available.

The reverse has been the case in America where in the sixties menopausal women accepted hormone treatment with increasing enthusiasm. In many cases this was overused. The effect of hormone treatment on the hair and the skin was soon noted and exploited, and the hormone oestrogen came to be regarded as an elixir of youth and a panacea for the many troubles that advancing age brings in its train, rather than as treatment of a deficiency.

The message arrived in Britain in the seventies. Here, the benefits of hormone replacement, as it was inaccurately called, were at first more readily recognized by journalists than by doctors. Then, thanks to the enthusiasm of crusading journalists like Wendy Cooper, many doctors in Britain and their patients began to realize for the first time the benefits of treatment.

In the mid-seventies, just as the wave of propaganda was resulting in much wider acceptance of the treatment, rumours of adverse effects, including cancer, spread from America to Europe. While the extent of the possible link remains unproven so far, some suspicions have been confirmed by research doctors. All powerful drugs can produce undesirable side effects, and hormones are no exception, particularly when improperly prescribed and taken. We now know that this has happened in certain instances in the past.

In treating menopausal distress every doctor will weigh the benefits for his or her patients against the possible risks. Restoration of hormone balance is not always as simple a matter as those who assert that it's just a question of overcoming medical ignorance or prejudice may believe. It would be wrong to lay down rules which take no account of individual circumstance. I have tried here to interpret the current medical and scientific thinking about the menopause, including that which remains controversial. Controversy is likely to persist until more results are known of the research which is being enthusiastically pursued in America and in the menopause clinics and research institutes of Britain. Already, as a result, safer treatment regimes are now being used.

The facts which are presented here should speak for themselves, showing that the benefits of treatment can more than outweigh any possible risks, *provided* certain essential provisions and conditions are fulfilled.

Barbara Evans, London 1978

# 1 Experiencing the climacteric
## What it is, and what it feels like

A wag has described a woman as a pair of ovaries attached to a body, and a man as a body which has two testes (sex glands), which may be only another way of repeating the old chestnut that women have a menopause, but men don't have a womenopause. In fact, men remain potentially fertile, and make and renew sperms throughout their lives. But when girls are born they already have all the eggs they are ever going to have, and when these run out at the menopause a woman's fertility is at an end.

The word 'menopause' has no derivative connection, of course, with 'men'. It comes from the Greek *menos* or month. Hence the 'monthly pause' or final cessation of the menses. The 'climacteric' or the years around the time when the menopause occurs, derives from the Greek *klimakterikos* or rung of the ladder. It can be taken as indicating that a stage of life has been attained.

The menopause is not purely a biological phenomenon. It is accompanied by psychological as well as physical effects which probably about 85% of women at the menopause notice as symptoms. The *climacteric syndrome* arises when these symptoms become complaints. This syndrome, which is discernible in about a quarter of all menopausal women, is more complex than it appeared to be when only hot flushing was equated with the menopause. We now know that it produces more esoteric symptoms than were formerly recognized. Unfortunately the distinction between symptoms which reflect, and are part of, the normal ageing of human beings and those which are superimposed on the ageing process cannot always be clearly drawn.

The first indication of the approach of the menopause is likely to be a change in the usual menstrual pattern. This may happen over a number of years, or the periods may cease abruptly and a menopausal woman may wonder if she could be

15

pregnant. In others the flow becomes more scanty, the intervals longer between each period and periods may be missed altogether. The character of the flow often changes, becoming paler, but it may be darker if, as sometimes happens, the periods get more profuse before menstruation finally comes to a halt. Abnormally heavy periods and flooding at this time should be medically investigated, and a woman should always consult a doctor if there is any bleeding between periods or after the menopause.

It is convenient to divide menopausal symptoms into vasomotor, genital, and psychological.


## 1 Vasomotor symptoms

Of all the troubles that women experience at the time of the menopause they complain most bitterly and most frequently about the hot flush. Flushing occurs when the nervous mechanism which controls the blood vessels is impaired and, in medical terminology, 'vasomotor instability' results. We all know people who are liable to blush more easily than others, especially when embarrassed or under stress. The blood vessels supplying the skin dilate readily in susceptible people, and this allows more blood freer access to the skin surface. About four out of every five women get some hot flushes at the climacteric. A Birmingham survey put the figure nearer 90%, while it was lower, at just over 55%, in a survey by the International Health Foundation (IHF). But this included women who had not yet reached the menopause. Flushing may come on a few years before menstruation actually stops, while a woman is premenopausal, and may be the first indication that the menopause is not far off.

Unlike some other symptoms experienced at the menopause, we know more about menopausal flushing because it lends itself to measurement. Women can keep an accurate note of the duration and the frequency of each flush, and this has provided us with useful information about the climacteric syndrome. For the study of other symptoms we have to rely on human memory, which may be affected by personal factors. Such studies are liable to be influenced by fear or hope, by suggestion, and by the psychological effect which the interest taken by a doctor often produces. At night, flushing disturbs sleep, and not only the sufferer's sleep, for her husband often gets a broken night when his wife gets up to change her nightwear, look for a towel, perhaps change the sheets and fling open the bedroom window. Women who get night sweats usually also get day sweats, some every few hours, some only a few times a day, or perhaps only once a day. The onset and duration of flushing is unpredictable but it is exacerbated by emotional factors, including anxiety or stress. The mild phraseology we often use may leave the uninformed under the impression that to flush is but a trifling inconvenience which soon passes. This is far from the truth. The sensation of warmth passes all over the body, the maximum heat usually being felt in the face and upper part of the chest, with patchy reddening of the skin in these parts. The shivering which follows may be equally unpleasant and is accompanied by sweating.

A number of women experience other vasomotor symptoms including palpitations and feelings of fright. Some describe a feeling of pins and needles in the skin or the sensation of ants creeping about over the skin (formication from the Latin *formica* – an ant) which can be disagreeable.

## 2 Genital symptoms

About one in ten women develop genital troubles which they often find more troublesome even than flushing. Genital problems arise because of loss of tone and elasticity and shrinkage in the passage from the womb (uterus) to the exterior (vagina) and from the bladder to the surface (urethra). These structures become unduly dry, and this may affect bladder and sexual functioning. In atrophic vaginitis, which until quite recently was known as 'senile vaginitis', a pejorative term indeed when applied to women as young as 45 or 50, the vagina loses its texture, becomes smoother and thinner and its cells suffer from loss of a carbohydrate substance called glycogen. This, in turn, leads to a reduction of the protective secretion of acid, so predisposing the thinned vaginal lining to infection; a resulting blood-stained discharge is not an uncommon finding at the climacteric. Pruritus, or itching of skin around the vaginal opening, can also be troublesome, even maddening.

In addition, as the vagina becomes less well lubricated, more sore, and less distensible, sexual intercourse becomes increasingly difficult, and is often painful. This condition, known as 'dyspareunia', due to vaginal shrinkage and atrophy may, if severe, make penetration impossible. The urethra is subject to the same atrophic change as the vagina, and this may also affect the sensitive base of the bladder. Passing urine becomes painful and frequent, especially at night when the urethra and bladder seem unduly irritable. By day a full bladder can cause stress or urge incontinence, exaggerated by laxity of the supporting tissues including the sphincters which control and close the orifices. A few women report an increase in sexual desire or libido caused by the irritation of the clitoris – the female counterpart of the male penis – due to the dry and brittle state of the vaginal lining and perineal area. The itching and scaliness of the perineal skin may contribute to the discomfort.

## 3 Phychological symptoms

Apart from the genital conditions which, like vasomotor symptoms, are diagnostic of ovarian failure, other symptoms may trouble women at the climacteric. I have grouped them under the heading 'psychological', for want of a more comprehensible term. This should not be taken to imply that they are part of a psychological disorder, but that a physical background cannot necessarily be readily identified, although the symptoms are real enough.

Women questioned by the International Health Foundation put their non-genital symptoms in the order shown below:

| Hot flushes | 55% | Dizziness | 24% |
| Tiredness | 43% | Palpitations | 24% |

| | | | |
|---|---|---|---|
| Nervousness | 41% | Lassitude | 22% |
| Excessive sweating | 39% | Pins and needles | 22% |
| Headaches | 38% | Muscle pains | 21% |
| Sleeplessness | 32% | Breathlessness | 18% |
| Depression | 30% | Impatience | 16% |
| Irritability | 23% | Other complaints | 11% |
| Joint pains | 25% | | |

A word of caution here. It must not be assumed that all these symptoms were necessarily due to the menopause. A psychiatrist would put many of them down to depression. A rheumatologist would see in the list many symptoms of rheumatoid arthritis. The menopause coincides with a period of life when stresses and domestic problems mount, and cause problems which are unrelated to the menopause. In addition, a number of the non-genital symptoms listed above are associated with each other, or with the genital conditions, and may be improved when the primary condition responds to treatment. A woman who gets up several times to pass water can hardly be having a good restful night. She will not wake refreshed in the morning if her sleep has been disturbed by finding herself in a sweat. An unsatisfied and unsatisfying sexual episode will further add to the irritable state in which she may eventually start the morning. No wonder she complains of lassitude. No wonder as the day approaches she feels both apprehensive and nervous, for soon the flush will return to distress her still further. Her head aches, she wonders how she will get through the day with its many tasks ahead. She can't remember exactly what she has to do, what she left undone yesterday. More palpitations, more anxiety, more irritability, as all the little household chores loom upon her, all yesterday's worries at work recur. Arguments with the family follow as they too rush about looking for the books and papers they *know* she must have moved. The hurried goodbyes, the general misery leave her in a state of gloom. She is now labelled 'depressed' and, indeed, she feels depressed and lacking the energy to cope with it.

The picture is a familiar one, the chain of events inexorably recurring. Women in an extensive study in Holland complained of symptoms similar to those mentioned in the IHF survey. This Dutch study involved over 6,000 women aged between 40 and 60, from a mixed rural and urban district, who answered a questionnaire about their symptoms. Besides the classical vasomotor symptoms, tiredness, nervousness, headaches, irritability, sleeplessness and depression were also frequently mentioned. Alteration in the normal menstrual pattern accompanied by infertility, and most instances of genital atrophy, were accepted by all the women; they were only mentioned as a complaint when the bleeding was abnormally heavy. The non-genital symptoms varied from one woman to another in severity as well as frequency.

By taking the menstrual pattern as a basis for analysis of these complaints, Dr L. J. Benedek Jaszman, head of the Department of Obstetrics and Gynaecology of the Regional Protestant Hospital at Bennekom, who conducted the study, has offered a rational explanation for many of the complaints noted among the women who answered the Dutch questionnaire. A pattern of events could be seen in their occurrence when these were evaluated, not according to the woman's chronological age, but according to her biological age, as measured by an index related to whether the periods were still regular, irregular or had ceased. Dr Jaszman established that tiredness, nervousness, headaches, irritability, dizziness and, to a lesser degree, depression, began to appear some time before the actual menopause, when the periods had become irregular in the previous year. The incidence of all these complaints rose increasingly as the actual menopause approached. He therefore attributed these symptoms to the early disturbance in the endocrine or ductless gland system. Ovarian function was still present, although diminished. The changes were attributable to the general hormonal imbalance which may and often does have psychosomatic undertones.

After the menopause, when the periods had ceased, the pattern of the women's complaints changed. They now most frequently reported the onset of hot flushes, perspiraion, formication, and pains in muscles, bones and joints, as well as sleeplessness, palpitations and dizziness. Sleeplessness showed a special pattern, and was most often reported by women who were five to ten years past the menopause; palpitations too were likely to persist, this possibly not being a menopausal symptom, but one found in the normal course of events as women become older.

By correlating the various symptoms which the Dutch women noticed, it appeared that hormonal balance was usually not restored until some five years after the menopause. This study was not concerned with genital symptoms, the women not being asked about these, but recently it has become clear that genital manifestations are more severe and last longer than has been realized. Women may admit to dyspareunia when questioned directly, but why should they have attributed this to the menopause? Like vaginal discharge it may not have been considered a suitably lady-like complaint to discuss with (predominantly) male doctors.

The Dutch women's complaints of aches and pains in the joints and bones were among the later symptoms they experienced at the climacteric, i.e. predominantly two or three years after the menopause. A quarter of the women who replied to the IHF questionnaire mentioned them. This symptom may be associated with the tendency for bones to become more brittle at this period of life. The end result, osteoporosis, is considered in Chapter 6.

### The premenopause

It is not generally appreciated how often symptoms arise before the periods stop. These 'premenopausal' symptoms come on insidiously and can be very severe without a woman realizing they are due to the approaching menopause. They are often not attributed to the menopause or recognized by her doctor if she mentions them because she is still menstruating, and in addition she may not have experienced the hot flush. More often her symptoms include characteristic increased irritability, with changes of mood and loss of libido, associated with the pain and dryness during sexual intercourse.

Such premenopausal conditions are more troublesome and

occur more frequently than many doctors have recognized in the past. Indeed they have not been studied in any detail and we have little information as to their frequency apart from the studies already mentioned, but there is no doubt about their occurrence or the distress they may cause, especially if they are overlooked – as may happen all too easily – and so left untreated.

Gynaecologist, John Studd, and his colleagues have reported (*The Menopause* 1977, edited by Robert B. Greenblatt and John Studd) that a fifth of the women among the first 300 who came to the menopause clinic at King's College Hospital, London fell into the premenopausal category. They were still having periods, but already had some typical menopausal symptoms. Most had asked their doctors to refer them to the menopause clinic, and most had previously been treated with tranquillizers or antidepressants. But less than half had had hot flushes. The majority complained of irritability (73.3%), depression (66.6%), poor concentration (60%), headaches (50%) and insomnia (45%).

It is interesting to find that certain symptoms are also more severe in the premenopause than after the actual menopause. The same team reviewed the records of 112 menopausal women whose main symptoms were hot flushing and sweating. In this group fewer women suffered from depression (50%), poor concentration (19%) or headaches (22%) than the premenopausal women.

By contrast, insomnia, which only 27% of premenopausal women suffered from, was reported by more menopausal women (38%), which bears out the impression that the night sweats and flushes are the main cause of sleeplessness. Dyspareunia was also commoner in the menopausal women than in the premenopause, as the vagina became increasingly atrophic.

Symptoms of climacteric may be:

---

**Genital:** atrophic vaginitis; urinary symptoms; painful intercourse.
**Extra-genital:** flushing and sweats; palpitations; dizziness.
**Early:** Hot flushes and sweats; atrophic vaginitis; urinary frequency.

**Late:** osteoporosis causing backache and pain; joint changes.
**Psychosocial, non-specific:** depression and irritability; insomnia; headache; loss of libido; anxiety.

# 2 Attitudes to the menopause

Over half the women who answered the questions posed by the International Health Foundation said they found the menopause psychologically upsetting. Two out of three French women agreed with this, and about the same proportion of British women. Of those who disagreed with the statement, the Germans found the menopause the least upsetting.

Menopausal women are often said to be difficult to live with, to have moods and to be unpredictable. The menopause comes at a time when many women are under pressure and already have much to contend with, but we have to remember that in the natural course of events depression is likely to increase rather than decrease with advancing years.

Our attitude towards the menopause is coloured by what we learned about it from our parents. Women were expected to be difficult and unreasonable in middle life, but they had to suffer in silence and put up with any inconvenience it might cause because it was the lot of women and in accordance with the laws of nature. Only time would help, but meanwhile no other help was available. Grandmothers and aunts had been difficult too. The situation provided an explanation for the peculiarities of awkward customers of which the world has its male as well as its female share, and not exclusively in the climacteric age bracket although psychological effects undoubtedly occur then. It is only natural for a woman to regret the end of an era if that era has been agreeable or to resent it if she has now no chance of improving a bad record. So to some it comes as a shock. Others find adjustment less difficult, future opportunities more promising, but in many instances a vicious circle develops all too easily, with the family reeling in dismay and helplessly unable to put a foot right.

Take the story of 50-year-old Evelyn whose marriage has

broken up. 'I saw my husband looking at me, and I could tell what he was thinking to himself; he was saying, "How old she looks." He could see what was happening to my skin and hair, and my waistline, and he was right of course. I *am* getting old, but so is he. I watched him looking in the glass himself. He too could see he was getting on.'

You have probably guessed the end of this story – a typical one which ends in different ways, but also begins differently in different women, and needless to say in different men – the pattern being set many years before the Evelyns of this world and their husbands reach middle life, even before they were teen-agers.

Throughout her childhood, Evelyn had lived in a middle-class conventional home, where her father came back every evening to an ordinary household, in which there was neither infidelity nor much evidence of warmth in her parents' relationship with each other. Her father was the one who bestowed the traditional kiss, and her mother the one who offered her cheek. It was not until her father died that her mother – at least in her daughter's eyes – demonstrated any evidence of affection for her late husband. By then it was too late. Shortly after this Evelyn, herself, married. Her mother had been conventionally pleased at the prospect of Evelyn's wedding and liked the prospective son-in-law but, nevertheless, in discussion one day, she admitted that she was sorry for anyone getting married. The ensuing conversation clarified the many hints which Evelyn had gathered as she grew up about her mother's dislike of the sexual aspects of her marriage.

Evelyn may not have been influenced by her mother's teaching, but during her own marriage she did not show any marked enthusiasm for sexual intercourse and was at times unwilling to accept her husband's approaches. He gradually adapted to her rejection and became, not impotent, but less active sexually, and the marriage rumbled on until, in its security and shelter, Evelyn's attitude to marriage and sex gradually warmed. By now, conditioned by years of apparent indifference to his advances, the husband was unable to respond. Evelyn then had what she considered a legitimate grievance. 'He doesn't care about me any longer.' And so we are back at the stage where in telling her story she said her husband realized they were both getting on in years. And she was 'menopausal'. And depressed.

Hormonal imbalance may cause changes in mood, excessive irritability or depressed feelings, and it is a well-documented fact that premenstrual tension, particularly in adolescents, can affect not only a girl's mood and behaviour but also her examination results and can even cause delinquency. It is estimated to cost 120 million working days a year in the United Kingdom. Our hormones or chemical messengers are powerful adjuncts without which we could not survive or reproduce the human race. No doubt they are responsible for much human success as well as failure, but their balance is easily disturbed both in adolescence and at the climacteric, which have many similarities.

So how justified is the charge of mental imbalance at the climacteric? It has been said many times that if men had a menopause we should know more about it now. As it is we have only in the last six or seven years begun to explore the labyrinth; and in the psychological field there has been a dearth of the research which is so much needed. There have been few well-documented and controlled studies into why women in middle life feel and behave as they do. We do not know nearly enough about the underlying causes of the symptoms, the influences which operate or why about one in five women suffer from depression at the climacteric.

### Environmental influences

A middle-aged woman has a multitude of reasons for finding that life has become more worrying than hitherto. The very fact that she may not feel able to cope with whatever problem is uppermost is a worry in itself. She may be worrying needlessly, but you can't necessarily stop worrying, even when you know already that it is counterproductive. We are, after all, living and breathing human beings who are affected by the other living and breathing human beings with whom our lot is cast. Let us look at the factors in a woman's life which can affect her psyche.

## 1 Her husband

By the time she has reached her middle forties a woman has probably had the same ball and chain for twenty or more years. Whether or not she and her husband love one another and have been faithful to one another, she is used to him, as he is to her. Both may have taken the other for granted; and ceased to notice changes in the other. In one survey 27% of husbands were unaware of the wife's menopausal problems. But if either is considering straying from the marital confines the husband is probably in a better position to do so than the wife, whose opportunities – if she wants them – are likely to be less than those of her husband.

She may not want to look elsewhere, but even if she does, she is likely to resent the fact that her husband has become more preoccupied with matters other than their sex life, or appears to be not at all preoccupied with her any longer. In fact, he may seem to have become lethargic where she is concerned. She may not have the insight to see that the years in which she so often rejected his approaches have taken their toll, leading him to reduce his demands in self-defence. She may now, like the Evelyns of this world, wish he were more responsive.

He is apt to be tired when he comes home, which gets later and later. Some nights he goes out as soon as the meal is over, or he settles down to the work he has brought back from the office. Or he falls asleep in front of the television set. He may wake grumpy, snap at his children and his wife, and subside with a glass of whisky.

If she stops to think, a menopausal woman may see that her husband's anxieties and responsibilities at work are heavier than before, with new partners, untried juniors, industrial troubles, and money worries building up. These factors, including possibly his wish to prove his potency with a younger woman, may be hidden from his wife, but none the less are possible explanations for the husband's withdrawn behaviour. The wife may well misinterpret his attitude and direct her own resentment at ageing against her husband.

As one menopausal woman said: 'I began to think my husband was menopausal himself. He was so irritable and impossible to live with. He was at the pub night after night, and if I went too it was always the younger people he wanted to talk to, not only the girls; it was the younger men that he seemed to like.' Eventually the husband changed his job, found other social openings and a younger partner.

After the divorce the wife had a few abortive affairs, but they did not satisfy her, and when she found a lover she would have liked to keep, her teenage daughter was critical of him, both to her mother and to the man, who eventually took off from his new abode. It is not surprising that the woman eventually presented herself at her doctor's surgery with depression.

## 2 Children

It is, unhappily, not necessary to be menopausal to fall out with your children. As they grow older they provoke their parents in different, but no less troubling, ways than when they were small. Increasingly they demonstrate their growing independence. *They* can escape at will, and, of course, do so but a mother is conditioned to care for them as long as they choose to remain in her house. Their acceptance of this situation differs from hers. The hotel syndrome usually emerges sooner or later, with the receptionist side of the mother feeling compelled not only to remain on duty but to include in her duties those of chambermaid, housekeeper, cook and washer-up. Old habits die hard.

The friends of her tenant children, who, incidentally, are often housed rent-free as well, often seem strange and unattractive. The ones that look as if they may be with the family for keeps as a son-in-law or daughter-in-law can all too readily assume the role of impostor in her eyes.

Sometimes the decision to leave home is taken because the son or daughter finds the mother too difficult to live with. This may be only too apparent, and will then be taken as another affront, indicating – as it may well do justifiably – that home conditions are unattractive. Two generations seldom cohabit without sparks flying periodically. The sparking episodes usually leave the mother more exhausted than they do the son or daughter, even if the husband has not, as may easily happen, taken the children's side of an argument. Maternal pride is now injured as well. With hindsight, or even at the time of an argument, a woman may be perfectly aware that she was in the wrong but still be unable to control her feelings or her words. Her sons and the young men who gather around her daughter may not show up her husband in too good a light either. Their youth is a constant reminder of her own advancing years, though this may be a subconscious reaction.

More serious worries may arise at this time, perhaps involving the police. Finding she has reared a drop-out, an addict or a girl who wants an abortion is another disaster she may have to face. The latter possibility may be particularly repugnant, and also confusing, to a woman who is herself having difficulty with her own sexuality. At the same time, a woman who has tried to adopt a liberal attitude to her daughter's sexual activity may find that her own spirit snaps. Out comes the phrase she would later dearly like to have bitten back: 'If you are old enough to make love you can surely do . . .' whatever the miscreant has failed to do for her mother.

Here all a mother's difficulties are with the very people she loves and has cherished. Where did she go wrong? she asks herself, losing even more confidence in the recollection. 'Don't worry about Mum,' the children say cheerfully to one another and to their friends. 'It's the change of life – a natural process after all. She'll get over it in time. She might be more cheerful tomorrow.' At other times, they are less charitable.

## 3 Parents

By the time a woman reaches the climacteric her own parents are more liable to have become frail and increasingly dependent on her. Their need for more active support not only complicates the lives of many women, but their emotional demands can be extremely exacting. The death of her own parents is another indication to a woman that her own youth has vanished, apart from the added feelings of loneliness which she experiences at the death of loved parents, and the final break with her old home.

## 4 Work and friends

At this stage in her life a woman with a job can expect to find it more tiring, partly because of her age and her commitments but also because, as seniority brings added responsibility, more is demanded of her. Fatigue is the enemy of good temper and this may make the menopausal woman less tolerant of the people with whom she works. They may respond by being less helpful than before. Moreover, new contemporary attitudes can disturb the older woman who has perhaps become less flexible in her outlook on life. Today's emphasis on the liberated woman may confuse those who have had less training and experience than men. Such a woman often feels inadequate and fearful of the future, and also guilty that she has not been as effective as the new generation of younger women now emerging vocally into a world where men have in the past been dominant.

Alternatively, a woman whose children are becoming independent may choose to return to work. She may have enjoyed her regular job before they were born, but to go back to work in later life is seldom as easy as it looks at first sight. There is the adjustment to a new discipline to be made as well as the physical effort of arriving on the job, especially if a woman wants to keep her house and home going as impeccably as previously. She may well find that, if she was bored before, now she has too much on her plate, and easily becomes overtired.

## 5 Looks and general health

Weight is a major problem in middle age. You cannot ignore the fact that a slim figure is more youthful-looking and attractive than an enlarged waistline. Skin and hair deteriorate with the years, and require more attention if their owner wants to look presentable; her wrinkles may discourage her, and, being no longer in the first flush of youth, clothes are less easy to find and usually more expensive. She is also only too aware that the rest of the world can see what is happening to her. Perhaps she herself knows that she is slowing down and is less effective. Now, although glad not to be pregnant, she may also wish that she had made better use of her opportunities for love and procreation, especially if she is childless, or regretting her lost youth. Life slips away and we forget 'it's always later than you think'.

As we know, about 85% of women experience some disturbance at the menopause. The symptoms in themselves can be worrying. Why is she so forgetful? a woman asks herself. She, who could always make up her own mind, now dithers. Why, suddenly, does she feel inefficient, more unpunctual, unable to finish a task? She even finds the car harder to park. Her headaches may be more frequent. She sleeps less well and is more jumpy and unpredictable. None of this is very serious, but it is upsetting and she asks herself uncomfortably if this is old age or just the dreaded menopause – or both?

## Psychosomatic symptoms

The emphasis then settles on the headaches and the insomnia. They are perfectly acceptable symptoms, and much less painful to dwell on than their underlying cause.

At this point the menopausal woman may ignore the real problem. She can now persuade herself that since she has a physical condition, this can be treated and will then go away. The picture which emerges is not that of a malingerer – the symptoms are real enough – but they reveal someone crying out for help. The doctor who listens to her string of minor complaints, including possibly palpitations, sees before him another middle-aged woman suffering from depression. Medical attitudes are mercifully changing, but once labelled a depressive, a patient is more than likely to be given antidepressants or tranquillizers, and it is possible for them to be repeatedly prescribed without reconsideration of the need or the effect.

She will label her doctor 'a very kind man, but . . .' and will resolve not to trouble him again when he is so busy. The pills don't help her anyway, but make her sleepy and less on the ball. So she stops taking them.

The same doctor may be perfectly correct in his diagnosis and treatment, and the patient's depression may not necessarily be associated with the cessation of the periods. Its roots may be buried in the past, and may possibly be related to separation from, or rejection by, her parents when she was a child. Disturbed early love relationships have far-reaching effects on subsequent relations with other people: husbands, children, or friends. They can alter a person's attitudes to the rest of the world for life.

Depression accounts for about half of all mental illness and is increasing steadily and rapidly, particularly in older people and in all walks of life. Apart from early life experience, some of us are more vulnerable than others, especially individuals with an obsessional personality, rather than those with a more happy-go-lucky outlook on life.

The typical depressive person is often tired, has a poor appetite and has usually lost weight. Though he or she may readily fall asleep, the depressive wakes frequently during the night and especially early in the morning, when life looks at its blackest. Tormenting thoughts recur during the hours of darkness with no prospect of any let-up. Feeling guilty, helpless and indecisive, the depressed person may be unable to face the daily task, or even the idea of going to work at all. At the extremes, many depressed sufferers express the wish to die, and a number of suicides occur among them. Symptoms gradually improve during the day and the cloud may lift, only to recur the following night. Changes in mood and drive are common in all of us, but the effect is exaggerated in the depressive, and a quarrel, a crisis or illness exacerbates the condition. Hence the confusion between cause and effect where the climacteric is involved.

Mental depression is commonest between the ages of 34 and 64 and occurs twice as frequently in women as in men. The distinction between depression arising within the personality, and that caused by the hormonal changes at the climacteric is often unclear. The psychiatric symptoms of anxiety, depression, irritability and swings of mood can readily be linked with the climacteric, but insomnia, apathy and loss of appetite can also occur for other reasons. Changes associated with ageing are meanwhile taking place and confuse the picture further.

In some primitive societies girls who had not begun to menstruate and women who had ceased to do so were treated rather as men, and took part in ceremonies from which women of child-bearing age were excluded. The menopause was considered of no importance apart from indicating the end of woman's sexual usefulness. Women in western societies have been at pains to disprove this fallacy, and to urge the retention of femininity well into advancing years.

Attitudes to the menopause vary from race to race, country to country and even between social classes. They frequently reflect the varying views about the role of women that prevail in different parts of the world. Where contraception is not practised the cessation of the periods is welcomed, or at least disregarded, by women in their forties who still have young children running around and needing care. They have no time to worry about the climacteric. In some developing countries there are women who are unaware that menopausal problems exist, but thousands of women elsewhere must have suffered uncomplainingly for generations, and it seems likely that there are still stoics who do not get help, and men who do not understand that they need it.

Lately we have had to think more carefully about the menopause and how to look after women with symptoms. Hormones are now used more widely than in the past and their greatly increased sales in Britain now place them in the fastest growing section of the pharmaceutical industry.

What has it been like for the women who have needed and been given treatment with these drugs at the climacteric?

*Elizabeth*
Let us take as an example, Elizabeth, now in her late forties, who has two daughters and a husband in business. She too worked in the business until a few years ago, when her elder

daughter took over her mother's job, and has made a success of it. Here is her story:

'I felt really dreadful and so limp I could hardly put one foot in front of the other. It was an effort to do anything at all, even to get out of a chair. I'm not a lazy person at all, but there came a time when I felt I couldn't get out of bed. I could have stayed there for weeks on end, and I was so depressed.' Looking back, Elizabeth thinks that depression may have been the first symptom. It was certainly severe.

She was then in her early forties, and after a while she went to see her family doctor. She told him she was fed up and found life altogether too much, what with her job, coping with her teenage daughters and their problems, and keeping the home going. She got, as many before her and since, sympathy, anti-depressants and tranquillizers, and instructions to take a holiday. She took the holiday, but not the drugs – at any rate not for long. They only made her feel worse, as she says, 'completely dopey all day. I'd fall asleep in the kitchen.'

For a year or so she just muddled through, and in retrospect wonders how she managed to keep going. Previously she had always had heavy periods and now they became irregular and infrequent.

Then came what she calls 'the real symptoms', easily recognizable as the hot flush. 'And a hot flush is not just feeling hot, you get a nasty feeling of faintness before the perspiration begins.' Apart from being bothered by the flushes, the faintness frightened her, particularly when she was driving her car. 'You get a strange feeling in your head and you know the flush is coming. It lasts a long time and leaves you feeling dripping wet all over, literally soaking. I'm a very fastidious person and I couldn't bear it. I was changing my clothes the whole time, practically living in the bathroom, and as fast as I changed them I was still wringing wet. At night I'd wake up in an unbearable sweat and just didn't know how to cool off.' Sometimes she would change her sheets more than once in a night.

It was also embarrassing. She got to the stage when she hated going to the hairdresser. 'When he touched my neck I knew it felt wet and clammy – terribly embarrassing. I imagined everyone was looking at me and could see all the sweat pouring off me, and my clothes clinging to my skin.'

Then she began to get headaches which Elizabeth thinks were even worse than the flushes, and were so severe that they used to wake her at night. Intercourse became difficult and painful and her vagina was dry. Her husband was kind but, as she said, 'the drive goes'.

Life became one long misery for her until one day she saw a television programme in which every one of her symptoms was mentioned. She didn't go back to her own doctor, whom she describes as 'very much of the old school, you've-got-to-get-on-with-it-dear type', but was fortunate in finding a woman doctor who had been at the receiving end of the climacteric herself. She thought at first Elizabeth looked too young to be menopausal but decided, having listened to her, that she certainly was.

The end result is that, after a thorough examination, Elizabeth has had treatment with oestrogen. If she stops the treatment her symptoms recur, but recede when she goes back on oestrogen.

Now that her symptoms have been relieved, what does Elizabeth herself think about it all? 'With hindsight you realize why you have been feeling grotty for years. But when you know it's the menopause it's like a psychological blow on the head. You feel your youth has gone. Womanly pride comes into it. Now you're middle-aged, and the knowledge that you are no longer able to reproduce has a psychological effect. It finally registers. I imagine it's like when you've had a hysterectomy.'

Of course, Elizabeth is not her real name. After she had agreed to tell me her story she stopped to wonder why anonymity was important to her, and why she did not want to be recognized by you who are reading about her. With delightful honesty she came to the conclusion that it was all a matter of vanity. 'I'm only 48, but if you admit to the menopause, everyone thinks you are over 50. I don't want to be old and no longer attractive. That's it – just a question of vanity.' She added, re-

flectively, 'I've a friend who doesn't mind admitting she's menopausal at all, but I do, and I'm resentful it came on me so early.'

It's a pity you cannot see how pretty, slim and attractive
Elizabeth is, for all she is 'menopausal'. To look at her and to
talk to her she could be much nearer 40 than 50. In addition to
relieving her symptoms she found the treatment improved the
condition of her skin and hair, though this may, in part, be due
to her feeling better. Her friends keep saying, 'You do look
nice,' – men too. Now that she is sometimes again subjected to
wolf-whistles she is not always certain how to react, and says
she had almost forgotten how to.

Technically, Elizabeth is not 'menopausal', since the word
'menopause' means only the cessation of the menses. She was
still menstruating when her symptoms started and they should
therefore be described as 'premenopausal' at the beginning of
the 'climacteric', which has been taken to cover a period of
several years, even twenty in some women, during which a
woman's life changes from the reproductive to the non-repro-
ductive phase. Elizabeth may still be ovulating, i.e. shedding an
egg between each period, and she has been told by her gynaecologist to continue to use contraceptives. In fact, symptoms
come on before the periods have stopped in about one woman
in five.

## Joan

Elizabeth is unfortunate in that the symptoms of the climacteric
came on so early. Joan – that isn't her real name either – is postmenopausal. In her case the menopause happened silently and
without warning when she was 50, and at first she thought she
might be pregnant. Seven years after her periods had stopped,
years in which she had no other symptoms, she began to wake
up night after night with splitting headaches. She describes
them as being 'as if my skull was going to pieces'. She could do
nothing about them, or about the accompanying insomnia,
which also appeared out of the blue, and was not affected by
sleeping pills.

She then found that she had to get up four or five times a

night to pass water. Her headaches would go after breakfast and perhaps after taking an aspirin, only to recur the following night. Joan was spared hot flushes, but did notice that on entering a room it would seem unbearably hot, and she wanted to fling open the windows. Where previously she liked a rather warm environment now she began to prefer cotton to woollen clothing. She too found sexual intercourse became uncomfortable unless she applied a lubricant jelly, of the type she had used previously as a contraceptive. All her symptoms disappeared when a gynaecologist prescribed oestrogen. Like Elizabeth, Joan too wishes she knew for how long she must continue treatment. Like Elizabeth, her symptoms which disappear completely on treatment recur immediately she stops taking her pills. The symptoms which both experienced are the cardinal indications of oestrogen deficiency – hot flushes, and thinning of the lining of the vagina with loss of elasticity, which causes painful intercourse and is associated with changes in the urinary passage. Other symptoms are often related to these two primary conditions. But no two women are alike, and all react individually. The menopause is very much an individual affair.

A third woman, well known to me, illustrates the other end of the spectrum, almost that seen in primitive societies where the reproductive period of life merges imperceptibly into the menopause: children are born, the pregnancy is followed by lactation; the hormones settle, pregnancy recurs, followed again by lactation. Life goes on in a regular cycle of events. The woman to whom I am referring had her last child at the age of 44. An easy confinement, and an uneventful recovery were followed on the tenth day after the birth by one massive loss of blood. Thereafter she had no further periods. She went back to work, and her friends said she looked rejuvenated by the last reproductive experience of her life. For her the menopause went by unnoticed, unrecorded and unlamented.

In most industrial societies the menopause occurs at around the age of 50 to 51 but single women or those who have never married may have an earlier menopause, which is difficult to explain. Environmental factors appear to have no effect on the age at onset, nor does education, physical type, the age at which the first period took place, the number of children women have had, their age when they were last pregnant, or their use of the contraceptive pill.

However, women of European extraction tend towards a later menopause. This may be associated with their state of nutrition. In New Guinea, for instance, a survey in 1973 among Melanesian women found the average age among the mal-nourished was 43.6 years. In those who were not considered to be undernourished the age was 47.3. The effect of poor nutrition may also be reflected in the low age of 44 years noted in 1966 among Asian women in the Punjab. Studies in America have suggested that thinner women have an earlier menopause, and some investigators have associated a higher income, or high social class, with a later menopause.

At whatever age they experience the menopause women who are not of European extraction complain less and appear to suffer least from the effects of the menopause. All women experience it, and about one in seven sail through it apparently undisturbed. Those who find it the least troublesome are those whose periods first started late, who have either never married or never been pregnant, and women who had a child when they were over 40. Women in the higher-income groups and the better educated have also reported fewer difficulties. On the other hand, women who have been bothered by premenstrual tension and the accompanying physical upset appear likely to find the menopause also troublesome.

## Premature menopause

For no obvious reason some women stop menstruating earlier than at the normal age, perhaps in their twenties. They often experience more troublesome symptoms than women at the typical normal menopause. A premature menopause may induce more backache and more tiredness. There may be more flushing which is often more persistent, and anxiety may be greater than at the usual menopause. Their condition may be associated with hormonal imbalance which can be rectified, or it may be caused by emotional factors.

## Artificial menopause

It may be necessary to remove ovaries because they are diseased, thus bringing about an artificial or surgical menopause. The symptoms of ovarian deficiency may then appear in a woman under the age of 40 even before she has left hospital after the operation. Subsequently her symptoms are likely to be more severe than at the normal menopause, with more persistent flushing, more joint pains, and severer depression than women who go gradually through a normal menopause. Her symptoms may also differ in certain other respects; for instance, in one study, sexual problems were found to be twice as common after an artificial menopause when compared with those of women of the same natural biological menopausal age.

A woman may occasionally slide imperceptibly into a menopausal state after hysterectomy or it may come on immediately after the operation even if the ovaries have not been removed. Here the symptoms of new psychological and sexual difficulties may be missed or not regarded as significant because, without her uterus, a woman now has no periods to indicate a menopausal effect.

As reported by John Studd, among 100 women whose ovaries were removed during hysterectomy before the menopause, hospital records indicated that over half the women had at least twenty-five flushes a day after the operation, the flushes coming on while 53 women were still in hospital. In 84 women they came on within six months of the operation, and in 32 they persisted for over a year. The commonest symptom which the women reported when interviewed in the menopause clinic between one and thirteen years after surgery was depression. Then came insomnia followed by loss of libido. It is significant that by then 34 women had no symptoms at all and although most women had hot flushes after the operation, only 28 had them by the time they were interviewed. Details are shown in the table.

Presenting symptoms in 100 women
1-5 years after removal of ovaries

| Symptoms | Numbers |
| --- | --- |
| Hot flushes and night sweats | 28 |
| Depression | 62 |
| Dyspareunia | 38 |
| Loss of libido | 46 |
| Insomnia | 48 |
| Headache | 32 |
| Aches and pains | 36 |
| Loss of concentration | 41 |
| Irritability | 36 |
| No symptoms | 34 |

From *The Menopause* (Clinics in Obstetrics and Gynaecology, Vol 4, No 1), guest editors Robert B. Greenblatt and John Studd.

Castration, which has such unpleasant connotations in connection with the removal of the testes in men, is now applied to the removal of the ovaries, a sad operation for a woman to undergo.

Amanda is an attractive producer in her early thirties who now has only a small part of one ovary left (probably by now functionless), having developed recurring cysts in both ovaries. This necessitated several operations, the first when she was 22. As a result, although the surgeon tried to conserve what ovarian tissue he could, she has been left in a state of almost complete oestrogen deprivation due to her artificial menopause. Her first flush came on soon after her last operation.

She admits to having previously regarded hot flushes as a joke. 'When people of my generation talk about them they fall about laughing. I remember giggling about menopausal women and their hot flushes, but when I had them I knew they were no joke.'

In spite of her first operation when parts of both ovaries

were removed she managed to get pregnant and after the baby was born her periods returned to normal. Then more cysts developed. She had another operation, and after this she failed to get pregnant again. Her periods became irregular and then stopped altogether, and in spite of hormone treatment, what was left of her one ovary failed to refunction.

She describes the hot flush: 'The first one came on suddenly when I was giving a dinner party. I felt a rush of blood to my legs and also over my shoulder and the top of my arms. It literally felt as if somebody was pouring liquid over me, and was very uncomfortable.' After the flush had gone, beads of sweat would break out on her forehead and her hands used to get very sticky. The flush would always come on in the same way, without warning, and spread over to her head, lasting about forty-five seconds. The only relief she could get was to go out into the cold air, though this didn't stop the flush.

When she first experienced her flushes they were coupled with the disappointing knowledge that obviously she was never going to be able to have another child. They were happening as many as five times an evening. 'Sleeping in bed was absolutely impossible, or any sort of normal married life, because I just used to boil up under the bedclothes and had to kick all the blankets off. And then as soon as the hot flush had gone I'd cool down and be freezing. It was very disturbing.'

She was attending the endocrine department of a big hospital, and had had various tests done before she was put on oestrogen. Her flushes disappeared in four days after beginning treatment.

She says she feels all right, but 'I'd expected to feel really wonderful like they tell you oestrogen makes you feel. Your hair's going to shine and you're going to be marvellous. But it was like the promised land. I don't feel incredible and I'm still more tired than I used to be, though I don't feel a creeping middle age as I did.'

I asked Amanda if she thought she had been affected psychologically. 'No,' she said. 'It's easier for me to accept what's happening to me at 30 than it is for somebody older. I *am* still young. I still *do* look young. I don't feel it's combined with the coming to the end of my attractiveness – I know it's the menopause. I'm not suffering under any delusions that it's not. But while it's tragic that we won't have any more children and want them very badly, I feel I'm lucky to have it now. At least I'm getting it over and done with. I've seen so many people who have such problems with the menopause – my mother's friends and the mothers of my friends, who've had great difficulty in dealing with the menopause.

'What *is* disquieting is that it's a life sentence; I know at 30 that I've to take hormone pills every day, perhaps, for the rest of my life.'

# 3 The structure and function of the reproductive organs

**The physiology of fertility and its termination**

You can see from the personal accounts of the climacteric in the last chapter that the symptoms vary from one individual to another. Why? And why do they occur at all? They are primarily due, as I have said, to the declining function of the ovary to which all women react differently.

The ovaries are the female gonads or sex glands. There are two, each about the size of an almond. They lie in the cavity of the pelvis or hip girdle, one on either side of the uterus or womb, and consist of fibrous and specialized hormone-producing tissue and egg cells. The latter make the essential hormones, oestrogen and progesterone. Each egg cell is contained in an envelope of fluid forming a follicle. The ovaries contain at birth several hundred thousand egg cells, all they are ever going to make during their lifetime. Many shrink and disappear, but around the age of 40 there are still many thousand eggs left in the ovaries which are by then shrinking themselves. During the reproductive period of life one egg matures every month and is released from the ovary, the process being known as ovulation. This takes place about the fourteenth or fifteenth day of the menstrual cycle and is accompanied by a slight rise in body temperature.

Each ovary lies just below one of the two Fallopian tubes (named after the Italian anatomist Gabriel Fallopius who described them). The egg or ovum, now half the size of a pinhead, passes through a funnel-shaped opening down this tube, which leads into the womb (uterus). Should the egg meet and be fertilized on its way down by a sperm swimming up the tube, pregnancy results. If not fertilized, the egg passes to the exterior in the menstrual flow.

The uterus, or womb, is a hollow muscular structure normally about the size and shape of a pear. Each of the two Fallopian tubes joins the upper part of each side of the uterus at its widest

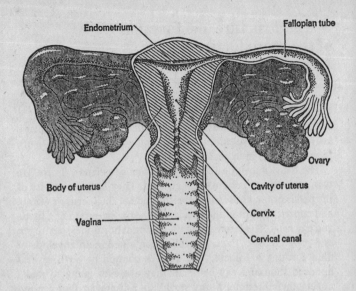

The female reproductive organs

part, where, in the event of pregnancy, the fertilized egg would implant, develop and grow, inside the lining, into a baby.

The lower part of the uterus, known as the cervix, is a narrow canal which leads down to, and projects into, the vagina through which sperms enter during sexual intercourse. The uterus lies in front of the rectum (the lower end of the gut) and behind the bladder.

The uterus is lined by a thick layer of cells and blood vessels, which comprise the endometrium. Under hormonal influence, the cells of the endometrium and its glands proliferate and it thickens in preparation to receive a fertilized egg. If none arrives, the endometrium undergoes a change in its glandular structure which becomes 'secretory' and is extruded as menstrual flow on the last day of the cycle, carrying with it the un-

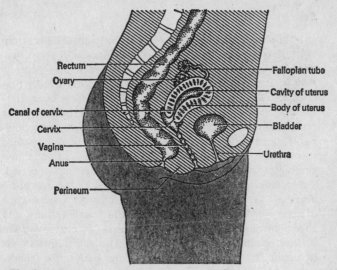

The female pelvic organs

fertilized egg; the whole process of the menstrual cycle is then repeated.

The vagina is situated between the rectum and the urethra (the passage leading from the bladder to the exterior). The area in which the vagina and the urethra open on to the skin surface constitutes the perineum. These structures have the same embryological origin.

The vagina also has its own lining and this too is under hormonal control. The cells which maintain its nutrition and lubrication alter according to the amount of circulating oestrogen, bringing about changes in these cells, known loosely as 'oestrogenization'. Microscopical examination of the vaginal smear provides some indication of deficiency or otherwise of oestrogen. (This is the basis of a test known as determination of the Maturation or Karyopyknotic Index, see page 108). Both the lining of the vagina and that of the urethra are related in structure and origin, and lack of oestrogen affects each similarly.

45

## Fertility

In all species fertility declines with age, but woman differs from animals in that her fertility is arrested when she is about two-thirds through her life or about thirty years after puberty. Animals retain fertility until death, though they usually produce increasingly smaller litters. Woman begins to be less fertile from five to ten years before the advent of the menopause provides clear evidence of the end of her ability to have children. Though the later menstrual cycles may not be accompanied by ovulation, doctors usually advise women to continue to use contraceptives until two years have passed since the last period.

Successful pregnancy has been recorded at the age of 57 years and 129 days (*Guinness Book of Records*). Over the age of about 40, there is a marked decline in female fertility, and once a woman has reached 50 the chances of conception are between one in 20,000 to one in 60,000. Available statistics show that male fertility declines ten years later than in the female, but, as I have said, whereas the female runs out of eggs at the climacteric the human male continues to make sperms into extreme old age, though the total number of sperms diminishes as the testes begin to degenerate. The relationship between the ovaries and the end of fertility at the menopause was realized in France at the end of the last century when extracts of animal ovaries were given by injection to older women with some reported success. The first natural oestrogen was isolated chemically in 1923, and others in 1930, but they were not suitable for general use in treating menopausal symptoms, being comparatively inactive when taken by mouth. They had to be given either by injection under the skin in diluted alcohol or oil, or as an implant. In 1938 the synthetic, stilboestrol, was formulated in England. It was more potent than natural oestrogens, although of a different formula, and could be taken by mouth.

Stilboestrol, prepared commercially in 1941, was then given for the treatment of menopausal symptoms on a rather hit-and-miss basis, in the absence of the knowledge we have today. It produced side effects that were at times as distressing as the symptoms it was intended to cure, namely headaches, nausea,

46

vomiting and bleeding, and it fell from grace. Natural oestrogens from living tissues, which have since been introduced commercially as 'conjugates', linked with a carrier in preparations such as Premarin, Harmogen and Progynova, have the effect of increasing the natural oestrogens in the blood.

Synthetic oestrogens, made chemically, are coal-tar derivatives, and have a different formula from natural oestrogens which are steroid hormones. Semi-synthetic oestrogens are made by linking a synthetic with a natural oestrogen; they exert similar effects to natural oestrogens. Ethinyloestradiol is thus a derivative of a natural oestrogen, oestradiol, and mestranol is derived from ethinyloestradiol.

Before puberty small amounts of oestrogen are made in ovarian tissue which maintains a regular but low supply. Around the time of a girl's first period some egg cells in the ovary mature and take over the main production of oestrogen, which is then progressively stepped up to meet the changes which are taking place at the beginning of the reproductive phase of female life. At the later stage some oestrogen is made by ovarian tissue from a precursor, androstenedione, and from the male hormone, or androgen, testosterone.

Two hormones, (the gonadotrophins) are instrumental in bringing about the changes in the menstrual cycle. They are produced by the pituitary gland which lies at the base of the brain, and is itself linked with the hypothalamus, an adjacent area in the brain from which it receives messages. These messages are influenced by the emotions, by physical factors, such as light, nutrition, temperature and drugs, and also by the amount of circulating hormones, including oestrogen. The system resembles a telephone exchange, and, like a telephone exchange, has been known to break down, and to transmit or receive faulty messages, which is how some menstrual irregularities may occur.

When enough oestrogen has been produced there is a feedback of oestrogen from the ovaries to the pituitary; an enlarged follicle on the surface of the ovary then ruptures and releases its egg. The ruptured follicle subsequently turns into a small, waxy structure, which produces a second hormone, progesterone. Acting alone in the first half of the menstrual cycle, and together with progesterone in the second half, oestrogen then brings about changes in the lining of the uterus or endometrium which allow its cells to proliferate to receive the egg if it should be fertilized. It can then embed itself and be nourished by the increased blood supply. Should the egg not be fertilized, preparation for its development will not be needed and progesterone then alters the nature of the endometrium, consolidating the cells into a stage in which the lining can be discarded. This secretory stage begins about the fourteenth day of the cycle, when the levels of the gonadotrophins have fallen sharply, which stimulates the pituitary to make more, and the ovarian/pituitary cycle is once more set in motion.

Just as ovarian activity is stepped up at puberty so it declines at the menopause when the ovary at last runs out of eggs. The remaining follicles wither and produce less and less oestrogen. Progesterone is also reduced, the decline preceding that of oestrogen. Levels of gonadotrophins rise – often beginning to do so a year before the actual menopause – but they have increasingly less effect on the flagging ovaries. Ovarian function slows to a halt, ovulation no longer occurs, and the periods, perhaps after some irregularity, finally stop altogether.

Meanwhile, in the absence of the 'braking' effect of oestrogen on the pituitary, the pituitary gonadotrophins remain high. These raised levels confirm the onset of the menopause and are diagnostic of ovarian failure. The same thing happens when the ovaries are removed from premenopausal women and oestrogen levels fall following a surgical or artificial menopause. Equally, if the ovaries of premenopausal women are destroyed by irradiation there is an immediate rise in gonadotrophins and a reduction in circulating oestrogen. This is not discernible when the ovaries are removed in older women in whom postmenopausal levels are already low.

As well as from the ovary, oestrogens are made by conversion in the body fats of male hormone precursors from the adrenal gland and in large amounts by the placenta during pregnancy.

There are two adrenal glands, one on top of each kidney. In addition to male hormones they also make cortisone, necessary for healthy functioning of the body. Before the menopause the ovaries and the adrenals share about equally the production of the precursor androstenedione, already mentioned. After the menopause the adrenals supply 85%, and the ovaries only 15% of the total. Approximately a year after the menopause the concentration in the blood of the precursor and oestrogen is down to about a fifth of the original level, but testosterone does not fall until from two to five years later, and then only to 60% of the premenopausal level. There is, therefore, some provision by nature for the effects of the declining ovary. But the need for oestrogen can be greater than the supply as is so often found at the menopause.

## Effects of oestrogen

We have seen that oestrogen maintains the balance between the action of the pituitary on one hand and the various hormones under its control. By its action on the brain it ensures normal pituitary growth enabling the latter to make the secretions which act on the ductless glands. Oestrogen acts on the genital system, the skin, the skeleton and the breasts.

Let us look first at the genital effects:

*The ovary.* This produces low levels of oestrogen until puberty. Thereafter, at ovulation, oestrogen assists in the production of the other sex hormone progesterone through the action of the pituitary gland.

*The uterus.* Oestrogen is responsible for bringing about and controlling the changes in the lining, or endometrium, causing it to thicken and the glands to become actively proliferative in the first half of the menstrual cycle. After ovulation, in the second half of the cycle, acting with the hormone progesterone it causes the lining cells to alter to a secretory form. At the same time it keeps the muscle of the uterus and the ligaments which support it and the other pelvic organs in good condition. After the climacteric the uterus becomes smaller and more fibrous, and the ligaments holding it in position tend to become lax.

*The vagina.* The lining of the vagina is particularly susceptible to a good supply of oestrogen which ensures that enough lactic acid is produced to keep the lubricating fluid made by the cells sufficiently acid. Without oestrogen the lining cells become thin, dry, and liable to infection with bacteria. Just as changes in the vaginal lining reflect the stage of the menstrual cycle and the amount of oestrogen being produced, so the cells which form the uterine lining show whether the latter is at the proliferative or secretory stage, and whether ovulation has occurred. At the climacteric the vaginal wall becomes shorter and less muscular and its secretions diminish.

*Bladder and urethra.* As with the other pelvic organs, oestrogen helps to keep the muscles and ligaments in good order. Like the vaginal lining to which it is embryonically allied, the lining of the urethra, or mucosa, depends on adequate supplies of oestrogen. Like the vaginal cells, those which line the urethra become thin, brittle and poorly lubricated in the absence of oestrogen, so that the whole lining including that of the bladder is rendered irritable and infection-prone. After the menopause muscle tone declines and the supporting ligaments in the pelvis lose their elasticity. This may lead to rectal and vaginal prolapse and to urinary incontinence.

So you can see that oestrogen plays a big part in keeping the genital system in running order until such time as it is no longer required to exercise its reproductive function. It does this by participating in the nutrition of the cells which produce enzymes, and so maintains the right balance of chemical salts and water in the body.

Now for the effect of oestrogen on the skin and hair. Both sexes produce both male and female hormones, though in differing amounts. A certain amount of androgen, the male hormone, is thus made by the female. Oestrogen counteracts the masculinizing effect of the male hormones on the skin and hair, so that women do not grow beards, or become bald, and their skin remains thinner and more supple than does men's skin after puberty. Women in America, where the administration of oestrogens has been more extensive than in Britain, noticed that their skin and hair improved on taking oestrogens, though the effect of ageing in women when the elastic fibres in the skin decrease should be remembered. It is idle to postulate that oestrogen taken internally or applied as a cream can eliminate wrinkles.

Oestrogen is responsible for the development of the breasts at puberty, the changes in the nipples and darkening of their surrounding skin. It maintains the firmness and glandular function of the breasts thereafter. At the climacteric they lose this firmness as well as their shape. Nipples become smaller and less erectile and the fat disappears from the breast tissue. Hence the sagging breasts in older women.

As we shall see later, oestrogen exerts a significant influence on the skeleton. Both calcium and phosphorus are needed to maintain old bone and to make new bone. Oestrogen influences the balance of these two main salts and furthermore supports the cells which are engaged in making new bone.

In spite of much controversy about the connection between oestrogen and depression, it is generally believed that oestrogen is a mental tonic, and almost certainly has psychological effects. It has other subtle actions of which we know little as yet. Too little. For example, women can smell certain musky odours which men, or girls who have not reached puberty, cannot smell. Postmenopausal women cannot smell them either unless they are being given oestrogens.

### Effects of progesterone

You will remember that progesterone is the other hormone besides oestrogen which is responsible for changes in the endometrium, and when acting in the second half of the menstrual cycle following ovulation, it alters the lining of the uterus to a secretory pattern. Progesterone acts only on tissues which have been previously subjected to the action of oestrogens. It in-

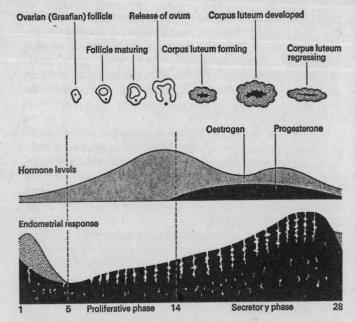

Development of ovarian follicle, production of ovarian hormones, and changes in endometrium during menstrual cycle.

creases the use of energy by the body and affects the amount of salt which the kidneys excrete. It causes few side effects but may make the skin greasy and may induce acne. It may also be responsible for breast tenderness and depression before the period.

Unlike oestrogen, progesterone is broken down by acid, and is rendered inactive in the stomach, so it is ineffective if taken by mouth. Consequently, soluble synthetic progesterones known as progestogens have been made in the laboratory, the main ones being norethisterone, which is chemically related to the male sex hormone testosterone, and norgestrel.

Progestogens may cause the bleeding between periods known

as 'break-through' bleeding, but when given in combination with oestrogens, progestogens effectively control heavy and irregular periods. Only one particular progestogen, dydrogesterone, does not prevent ovulation from occurring but other progestogens are widely used in combination with synthetic oestrogens in the contraceptive pill, when the main action is the prevention of ovulation.

Progesterone is assuming increasing importance since the discovery by scientists that it has the power to neutralize some of the effects of oestrogen. One action takes place within the cells of the endometrium themselves and blocks the accumulation of oestrogen there. Progesterone can also promote the formation of an enzyme which destroys oestrogen, so when given in conjunction it counteracts some undesirable effects of oestrogen.

# 4 The menopause and the psyche

About one in every two women have some disturbing psychological effects before the menopause. Life can, we know, turn sour for some women in middle life according to their temperament, and the circumstances in which they find themselves, and the development of 'the empty nest syndrome'. How much the depression which some women experience at this time is due to their dissatisfaction with their lot and how much to the hormonal imbalance or a combination of social and hormonal change is hard to determine. Oestrogen is certainly a mental tonic, and recent research suggests that the special mechanism by which oestrogen gains access to the nucleus of certain body cells may also operate in the brain. It may be that the withdrawal of the stimulus of oestrogen leaves the brain in a condition which contributes to the onset of depression in those who are predisposed, though this may be difficult to prove.

One way of investigating symptoms and response to treatment is known as the 'double-blind' trial. Here an inert substance, usually lactose, is given as a tablet for a period of time, and then a test preparation, which is identical in appearance, is substituted for the same length of time as the first substance or 'placebo'.

Alternatively, the test substance may be given first and then changed to the placebo. Those who agree to take part in, or to conduct, a double-blind trial are usually told that the tablets are of different strength or type but neither party knows the code which is to be used in interpreting the effects. The hope is that this will eliminate the influence of suggestion in assessing the results. It is not entirely foolproof and the findings may not be conclusive, because anyone who is receiving medical attention and interest may feel better, even while taking inert tablets, simply by the psychological uplift this gives. This is known as the 'placebo response', and it is remarkably common. A psychiatrist once said that every doctor is a 'walking placebo'. Even flushing, which we know is caused by ovarian deficiency, sometimes responds to a placebo. This was well demonstrated in some studies which were made at the Chelsea Hospital for Women, in which women who agreed to take part in two double-blind trials were either postmenopausal, or were at the stage where their periods were infrequent with at least three-monthly intervals between each period.

In one short study which lasted four months the women, who all had severe symptoms, were given a placebo for two months and this was replaced by oestrogen for the next two months. Women with milder symptoms cooperated in another trial which lasted for a year, during which they received a placebo for six months and then took oestrogen for six months. They filled in a questionnaire at the beginning and at two-monthly intervals during the trials.

In the shorter trial, both vaginal dryness and flushing improved on oestrogen, as would be expected, but some women

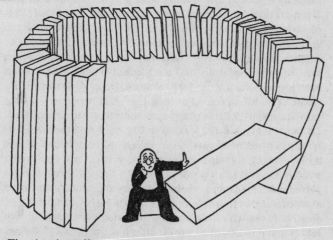

The domino effect

while they were taking the placebo (of which they were un-aware) also said their flushing and vaginal dryness disappeared. Insomnia, irritability, headaches, anxiety, frequency of passing water, memory, spirits, and optimism also improved. This might have been a domino effect, in which one symptom or situation affects another, another, and so on; but the same women also claimed their skin and appearance benefited from the placebo.

In the longer study the response to oestrogen was greater for flushing and vaginal dryness, as you would expect with longer-lasting treatment, but in this trial the placebo had a different effect from that in the shorter trial. It did *not* improve flushing or vaginal dryness although a number of women still main-tained their skin had improved. The results were unaffected by the order in which the placebo and oestrogen were given. This type of study is justifiable only when the symptoms are mild or, if they are severe, only for a short period of time. The other difficulty in assessing results arises with the immediate reap-pearance of the symptoms of hot flushes when the change is made to a placebo *after* taking oestrogen. Here the effect is so clear cut that the recipient is no longer in any doubt that she is receiving a placebo. Coincidental emotional or psychogenic symptoms then become harder to assess, or even impossible.

Some studies, however, have pointed to conclusions which are likely to be valid. In 1933 the Medical Women's Federation sent a questionnaire to 1,220 women from all walks of life whose periods had ceased at least five years previously, asking the nature and duration of any symptoms they had experienced. Of those who answered, just over 30% said that they had suf-fered from nervous instability, while 60% complained of hot flushes lasting for an average of two years. Only one in ten women had had to stop work or stay in bed. Of those who re-ported suffering from nervous instability the women who were married put this fourth in order after headaches, giddiness and obesity. Those who were not married rated nervous instability higher and put it third on the list after headaches and giddiness.

Another investigation has illustrated that women of different ages react differently to both physical and psychological troubles. In 1965 two Americans, Doctors B. L. Neugarten and R. J. Kraines compared the symptoms of 460 Chicago women aged between 13 and 65 years. Those between 45 and 54 years old were asked to rate themselves as premenopausal, menopausal, or postmenopausal. When analysing the reported symptoms the investigators found more physical symptoms in the group of menopausal women, and more psychological symptoms among the adolescents. There was little difference between the other groups in overall psychosomatic and psychological symptoms, except that these were significantly less in women aged 55 to 64 years and presumably postmenopausal. The physical symptoms which the menopausal group of women reported were predominantly flushing, sweating, aches, flooding and tingling sensations. But certain individual symptoms were more troublesome at the menopause, in particular nervous instability and irritability, which was reported by 92% of menopausal women, by 90% of young women aged 20 to 29, by 82% aged 35 to 44, by 76% aged 13 to 18, by 71% aged 45 to 54, who were not menopausal, and by 48% of women aged 55 to 64.

The two doctors attributed this increase in sensitivity to all symptoms and their increased frequency in adolescence and at the menopause to the changes which take place in the sex hormones at these two stages of life, which are comparable in some respects as times of hormonal change. When Dr Jaszman and his colleagues analysed the symptoms of women who took part in the Dutch inquiry they classified them according to the biological age, determined by their age in relation to menstrual changes, as opposed to the chronological age of the women who reported them. They then found that the symptoms fell into three distinct groups which occurred at identifiable times related to the three stages of the climacteric: premenopausal, those that arose before the periods had stopped, menopausal, those which arose around the time of the cessation of the periods, and those that were postmenopausal after the periods had already ceased. The three groups were:

1 Vasomotor symptoms, flushes and sweats.
2 Fatigue, headaches, irritability and depression.
3 Shortness of breath, palpitations, insomnia and mental imbalance.

The symptoms in the first group were usually experienced about two years after the periods had ceased when they would be due to established deficiency in the oestrogen supply. The second group of symptoms predominated earlier, while the periods were becoming irregular during the period of hormonal imbalance but some oestrogen was still being produced by the ovaries. This was particularly noticeable where irritability was mentioned. Of thirteen complaints listed by the Dutch women the only clear psychiatric symptom was irritability, which in the premenopausal women came fourth in frequency and in the menopausal women fifth. As for the symptoms in the third group – sleeplessness, breathlessness, palpitations and mental imbalance – these did not seem to be peculiar to the climacteric, and were unrelated to the changes in the periods. The general conclusion was that they should be regarded as part of the general effects of becoming older in the ordinary course of life.

Three English general practitioners have confirmed some of the Dutch findings. Doctors B. Thompson, S. A. Hart and D. Durno questioned all the women in their Aberdeen group practice aged between 40 and 60 in 1973. They found that 93% of their climacteric patients had experienced flushing, and that this was most common (as the Dutch found) in the first two years after the periods had ceased, but depression, the only psychiatric symptom which was specifically mentioned in the inquiry, could not be related to the climacteric.

While some doctors believe that oestrogen plays little or no part in psychiatric climacteric symptoms, Dr F.P. Rhoades, who studied 1,200 postmenopausal American women suffering from poor memory, depression and fatigue, which he regarded as psychiatric in origin, found that 95% improved during two years' treatment with oestrogen. In another smaller survey other American doctors, H. Lozman, A. L. Barlow and D. G. Levitt, obtained similar confirmation of Rhoades' findings.

58

For over thirty years British gynaecologists have used oestrogen for severe menopausal symptoms, but American doctors and their patients have been more enthusiastic in claiming its advantages, and have used it more widely than the British. At the same time the regimes in the two countries have differed as well as the dosage. This may account for the apparently conflicting evidence in the various investigations which have been done, and the greater volume of work which has been reported in America.

But British research is gaining momentum, and in Dundee a psychiatrist, Dr Barbara Ballinger, has been particularly interested in finding out more about the prevalence of psychiatric illness in the general population of women at the time of the climacteric. With the help of six general practitioners she sent a questionnaire to all women aged 40 to 55 years on their lists. She asked them to answer questions about their general health, their menstrual state, and their family situations. Her questions had been designed to detect mainly depressive and neurotic illness, and she tried to correlate their replies with evidence of psychiatric disorders.

She was surprised to find how many apparently normal women at that age should probably be regarded as psychiatric 'cases' without being seriously disturbed. Of 539 women a total of 155, or 29%, could be described as mildly psychiatric. They were not women who had taken any medical advice or considered themselves to be in need of help. They were simply on a doctor's list. She then investigated a number of women of the same age who *were* attending a doctor, though not necessarily for a menopausal condition. Among them she found a higher proportion, 55%, who could be considered to be psychiatrically affected. Finally, in a hospital gynaecological clinic she found that 55% of the patients who were attending for treatment of general gynaecological complaints were probably suffering from some form of psychiatric disability.

Dr Ballinger confirmed from the answers she had received that vasomotor symptoms – sweating and flushes – increase at the menopause. But although both vasomotor symptoms and

59

psychiatric illness were, according to her, related to the cessation of the periods, the relationship was not the same. Vasomotor symptoms increased dramatically when the periods stopped, and might continue for five years thereafter. But minor psychiatric illness usually began to increase earlier, before the periods had finally stopped, and commonly lasted only about a year.

Dr Ballinger's useful research has provided documented evidence of a considerable increase in minor psychiatric illness at the time of hormonal imbalance as the periods cease, which may persist for about a year.

Her findings are similar to those of Ben Moore, R. Gustafson and John Studd at the Birmingham and Midland Hospital for Women, where 55% of women seen in the menopause clinic were suffering from depression, 38% complained of insomnia and 30% of lethargy.

In Merthyr Tydfil Doctors M. Aylward and J. Maddock found an even higher proportion of psychiatric illness among a group of women picked at random, whose periods had ceased within the previous two years. Over half showed some features of mental depression, as classified in the table.

| | |
|---|---|
| Inability to make decisions | 79% |
| Apathy and inner unrest | 65% |
| Irritability and aggressiveness | 51% |
| Depressive thoughts | 47% |
| Disturbed sleep | 46% |
| Slowing of mental processes | 38% |
| Loss of libido | 37% |
| Loss of emotional reaction | 18% |

In recent years there has been speculation that alterations in body chemistry may play a part in depressive states at the time of the menopause. It is interesting that Dr Aylward has found associated changes in the role of a group of substances known as indoleamines in menopausal depression. One, tryptophan, circulates in the body attached to the blood proteins as a 'bound' form, and also as a 'free' unattached form. If the links are broken, bound tryptophan changes to the free form. Certain drugs, including oestrogen, have the power to release the binding links, changing bound to free tryptophan, an important effect, because free tryptophan probably influences the way the brain functions.

Dr Aylward was able to establish that the total blood tryptophan is lower than normal in women whose ovaries have been removed, and is also lower in depressed patients. By double-blind trials involving women without ovaries and those in whom they had not been removed, he was able to show that giving oestrogen effectively raised free tryptophan blood levels and improved the symptoms of depression. He proved that there is a significant correlation between reduced free tryptophan levels, low oestrogen and the severity of postmenopausal depressive illness.

In the USA, E. L. Klaiber had already found a biochemical link between depression and oestrogen deficiency, although he did not analyse the symptoms and did not measure the oestrogen blood levels. He was able, nevertheless, to report that 60% of severely depressed women improved significantly after three months' treatment with oestrogen. But they needed bigger doses – up to ten times – than were required to improve vaginal dryness, and the women who received early treatment were evidently more susceptible to it. Klaiber put forward the suggestion that severely depressed women may have become resistant to oestrogen.

This emphasizes the urgent need for more research into the biochemical changes in the body which take place at the climacteric. It would be particularly interesting to know why psychiatric symptoms when they arise at the climacteric usually precede the cessation of the periods.

**Effects of oestrogen on mental processes**

It is widely believed that oestrogens influence not only human behaviour, but mental functioning. However, in spite of strong indication of this possible effect, mental testing has so far failed to produce substantial evidence that giving oestrogen improves performance. In Finland Professor L. Rauramo compared 65 women whose ovaries had been removed at hysterectomy with a control group of women who had had only hysterectomy, some of whom were given oestrogen. Although Professor Rauramo could not prove by psychological testing that perceptive processes improved on oestrogen, emotional factors seemed to be affected. Women who were not taking oestrogen felt that without it their memories were poorer and their concentration and powers of attention were weaker.

In Belgium Doctors G. Vanhulle and R. Demol in double-blind trials in postmenopausal women found oestrogen had significant effects on mental functioning, and in West Germany Dr Gertrude Krüskemper, studying women who were asking for advice about losing weight, thought the premenopausal women were more stable than those who were postmenopausal. But much more investigation is needed to provide scientific proof of correlation between mental processes and the beneficial effect of oestrogen, apart from its accepted action as a psychological tonic.

The menopause does not appear to give rise to a specific pattern of psychological symptoms. In relation to the general increase with age of psychiatric illness in women, the effect of the menopause is relatively small, in spite of some conflicting reports. Admissions to mental hospitals increase with age in both sexes, but more steeply in women, with a peak in the climacteric age group, but there is no evidence to suggest that the menopause induces psychiatric illness or psychological changes apart from adding to the stress upon a woman already predisposed to anxiety and depression. The symptoms of oestrogen deficiency and of anxiety and depression are often mixed, and the relief of one may help the other.

As the French gynaecologist, M. Colombat de L'Isière, wrote as long ago as 1845: 'Like the first appearance, so the cessation of the periods varies in different subjects, and is in subordination to the temperament, the constitution, the climate and the habit of life of the female.'

# 5 Psychosexual aspects of the climacteric

Her fortieth birthday is a significant milestone for every woman although she may feel exactly as she did when she was 39 and 364 days old. She asks herself what she has done with her 40 years? Nothing? None of us, men or women, has done all we would like with our lives, but even if a woman's reproductive achievement has been considerable and she has reason to be content with her record she may still be aware that she has missed out on a particular slice of life.

This realization has a devastating effect on some women, who then embark on panic measures as they see time running out. They become more self-assertive, more thrusting and more ambitious. After all, they argue, soon I shall be old. Soon I shall be menopausal. As they determine to make up for lost time a number of women, often middle-class, behave in an uncharacteristic and unpredictable way. Although they have never previously even contemplated an extra-marital relationship and would be seriously wounded were their husbands to do so, now they proceed to the odd affair, as if in desperation to prove their power to themselves and possibly the world. At first it's amusing, then exciting, and finally absorbing. And though the woman has no wish to destroy her marriage or leave her children, the new relationship turns out to be more sexually rewarding than the one she has experienced with her husband. It is not as unusual as you might think for women to learn at this moment that they have never experienced a satisfactory orgasm within marriage and that they might have all this time enjoyed, in Katherine Whitehorn's apt phraseology, belonging to a 'two-orgasm family'.

Finding what she has missed all these years may have a far-reaching effect on a woman's attitude to the menopause, and, of course, to her husband. Whether the latter is aware of the reason for his wife's resentment or not, he is likely to lose his own confidence. His sexual performance with his wife may so deteriorate as to leave him impotent, or at least unable to meet all her demands. At the other end of the scale some women go totally off all sex at the climacteric. A woman may already have lost respect for her husband, while others may suddenly take an irrational dislike to their life-long partners. 'I cling to the edge of my side of the bed for fear I shall brush against him,' one woman said. And another said, 'I can't bear to kiss him when he comes home in the evening.' Yet both admitted they had no intention of knowingly allowing the man to find solace elsewhere. He might find the grass greener (and younger) on the other side of the fence – errant males *can* stay away for good and take their money with them.

Fortunately, loss of libido at the climacteric is transitory in many cases and can be helped by discussing the problem openly, and by reassurance from whoever is looking after a woman medically. It should not be ignored. The administration of hormones can be used if counselling fails to improve libido, and vaginal creams applied to treat soreness and pain.

It will be recalled that in her inquiry regarding the incidence of depressive illness in the general population, Dr Barbara Ballinger found an unexpectedly high proportion of women who had not sought medical aid, but who appeared to be suffering from psychiatric disturbance between the ages of 40 and 55. Dr Ballinger subsequently discussed their sexual relationships with 114 of these women who agreed to be interviewed. As might be expected she found that the happiness of the marriage affected the woman's sexual response. Of these 114 women, 34 said their sexual responsiveness had deteriorated and 5 said it had increased. 24 women had never enjoyed sexual intercourse and their attitude had not changed; 27 women found it satisfactory and it continued to be so; 5 women had refused to have sexual intercourse at all for from five to seventeen years. Of the 90 women who had husbands, 21 said the relationship was a poor one; in 25 it was described as fair and in 44 good. Only 40% of those women who had persistently poor libido or had experienced a recent deterioration in libido enjoyed good relations with their husbands while 66% of women who had *no* impairment of libido were happily married.

## Alteration in libido

Sexual interest and drive gradually decline with age in both sexes and a corresponding diminution of sexual activity follows. The usual method of measuring sexual activity by frequency of intercourse and of orgasm cannot be applied to women because, as Doctors E. Pfeiffer, A. Vervoerdt and G. C. Davis of Durham, North Carolina have indicated, when women stop having sexual intercourse they usually attribute this to lack of interest on the part of the husband; and men also assume the same thing. These American investigators therefore questioned men and women about their interest in sex rather than their sexual activity. Among the women aged 46 to 50 years, 7% expressed no interest in sex, and this figure rose to 51% by the age of 61 to 65 years. By contrast, the number of men who had no interest in sex rose only from 0% to 11% at the same ages, the sharpest change taking place between the ages of 45 and 55.

It has sometimes been said that some women become more sexually responsive in middle life, but in Sweden Dr Tore Hällström, professor of psychiatry in Gothenburg, investigated 800 women aged between 38 and 55, all of whom were living with a man, and found that sexual interest, capacity for orgasm and frequency of sexual intercourse showed a declining trend. Whatever their age, few women reported an increasing interest in sex as they got older. 63% of women aged 50, and 72% aged 54 said their libido had deteriorated.

Is the decline in women's sexual interest a consequence or a cause of less frequent sexual intercourse? Probably age is the commonest cause of failing sexual drive in men, but in the Swedish study although the women thought the decline in their sexual activity was due to this, in fact, whether or not the woman's interest had waned, the difference in their ages was the same between the men and women concerned, and reduced activity could not therefore be attributed to the age of the man.

Women whose interest in sex was reduced more often reported stronger desire in the man than in themselves, these findings supporting the conclusion that reduced sexual activity is more often a consequence than the cause of women's declining interest.

The part played by the climacteric is difficult to separate from the effect of ageing. Pfeiffer and Davis, on analysis, think the climacteric makes a small but significant contribution to sexual malfunction, but less than marital set-up and age.

In England, John Studd found that of 300 women who came to the menopause clinic, 96 had recently lost libido. They fell into two categories: 36 complained of dyspareunia with or without a change in sex drive, and also had atrophic changes in the vagina, and 60 had no vaginal atrophy, but loss of libido alone. 40 women in the second group had already been given oestrogen for this, but without effect, and there was no evidence from laboratory investigation that they were deficient in oestrogen. Libido improved only with the addition of androgens or male hormones. Here the results were remarkable in that 80% of women who initially had lost their libido found sex drive and enjoyment were restored by treatment to as good or better than before the menopause. In spite of this response John Studd and his colleagues at King's College Hospital could find no relationship after the climacteric between psychosexual symptoms and the amount of oestrogen or of testosterone in the blood before treatment. So the treatment cannot be straight replacement of a chemical deficiency.

The falling off in sex drive and interest in middle life is likely to be due to external factors induced by an upset in the endocrine system rather than to hormone deficiency. This view is supported by a Swedish study in which the amount of oestrogen in the urine of 146 menopausal women was measured, and appeared to be unrelated to their interest in sex. Sexual interest tails off more slowly in men than in women in later life. In the case of women this may be due to a number of possible factors including dyspareunia, the husband's health or lack of emotional warmth, or as a result of the passage of time. However, dyspareunia is not normally very common, except in the presence of atrophic vaginitis. Approximately 5% of women say they often experience it, only 2% consistently do so. Other factors are probably more closely related to loss of libido, such as social class, education and mental health. Depression is a more likely cause of lack of interest in sex than other forms of mental illness.

Then there is the attitude of women themselves. Those who are resigned to a lower quality of sex life will get this however frustrated and rebellious they may be inwardly. This negative female approach to sex will undoubtedly alter in the future, as more women advance along the path to liberation.

Changes in the capacity for orgasm and in sexual interest in women in any age group are already taking place. Dr Alex Comfort has frequently expressed the opinion that age need be no barrier to continued sexual experience, and that this is not only comforting but a prophylactic against the development of marital disharmony. According to him, people stop having sex for the same reasons they stop riding bicycles – general infirmity, thinking it looks ridiculous or having no bicycle. They should expect to enjoy sex long after they have abandoned their bicycles. As for looking ridiculous, in his view, making love doesn't look any sillier than, say, playing golf.

Kinsey has shown that ageing need not affect a woman's sexual capacity until late in her life; this is particularly the case when regular and effective sexual stimulation is continued.

As the Swedish workers indicated, the commonest cause of declining sexual activity is the falling off of interest on the part of women. Their deterioration in libido is often related to the pattern of sexuality established before the menopause. About 5% of men are impotent at the age of 45 and this rises to about 10% in the middle fifties. Loss of female libido may be husband-induced, in which case it would be wrong to attribute the cause of the wife's loss of libido to her menopausal state. For her own self-respect it is important for a woman to realize that her menopause may not be the cause of her husband's lack of interest. Nor does the onset of the menopause necessarily justify the fears of another woman in the husband's life which haunt so many women at the climacteric, and which may lead them in the wrong direction. There is no proof that the high proportion of divorces – nearly 40% – that involve middle-aged couples in the UK is a consequence of the climacteric, but only another indication of the pressures on women at this time.

## Sexual responsiveness in women after the menopause

It is commonly, but erroneously, held that women who are past the menopause cannot respond sexually. However, W. H. Masters, now director of the Reproductive Research Foundation, St Louis, Missouri, considers that 'given a reasonably healthy male as an interesting and interested partner there is no reason why effective sexual function can't continue for women into the 70 and 80-year-old group'. The fallacy about older women's sexual incapacity is engendered by the young who regard coital activity in their parents as incongruous if not ludicrous, and often appear unable to recognize the manner of their own beginning or begetting. Thus Hamlet to the Queen, his mother, speaking with disapproval of her sexuality: '. . . at your age, the heyday in the blood is tame'.

As in all forms of activity, where sex is concerned the more practised the performer, the more expert he or she becomes. The performance may be less frequent than in youth, but this could enhance the pleasure given and received. Few older women advertise their continuance of sexual activity because public opinion regards it as abnormal after the flush of youth has been replaced by the flushes of the menopause. Many doctors too readily accept this view. Male doctors are often ignorant of important aspects of female sexuality. Medical students, who incidentally are usually taught by men, have virtually no instruction in the subject.

## Effects of ageing on sexual function in men

Popular misconceptions about sexuality in later life are liable to affect an older man, who may then retreat from a sexual situation in which he fears he will fail because of his own inadequacy. He should understand that it is not shameful sometimes not to ejaculate into the vagina. This may be normal in older people, especially if intercourse takes place frequently. It may take an ageing man longer to ejaculate, but he does not have to do so every time he has intercourse. He is more likely to fail by trying too hard unless both partners accept this limitation. A man who does not choose to relax may continue a thrusting session which he feels he must pursue but which pleases neither partner. He is better advised to satisfy his own level of demand.

A man over 55 usually takes longer to achieve erection than a younger man. The onset of his ejaculatory process may be delayed, and the length of orgasm shortened. But the older man seldom experiences the pain that younger men get in the testes as a result of prolonged sexual foreplay without ejaculation, caused by the extra blood carried into the testes. A woman who understands these facts should be able to make allowances for, rather than demands on her sexual partner.

## Effects of ageing on sexual function in women

The sensitivity of the skin declines with age, and whereas premenopausal women may enjoy play with their breasts and nipples prior to sexual intercourse, in some women this stimulus loses its strength after the menopause, although general sensual awareness is not necessarily diminished. The normal response to genital stimulation can also be affected by atrophic vaginal and perineal skin changes which, if untreated, may result in shrinkage of the fold which protects the clitoris. The exposed clitoris is then liable to irritation by the scaliness of the surrounding skin, and perhaps to infection. Genital stimulation instead of causing enjoyment may then be painful and so unwelcome.

If, in addition, the lubrication of the vagina is reduced and if, at the same time, the vagina becomes less distensible it is harder for the man to penetrate the opening, and the woman may refuse intercourse because of the pain and difficulty encountered.

In older women the rate of lubrication normally engendered by sexual excitement is slower and its duration may be shorter, just as it takes longer for the older man to achieve erection. In this instance the woman may lubricate sufficiently to allow penetration, but not long enough to protect the thinned vagina from the amount of thrusting at coitus which it could hold in the premenopausal years.

Small slits or minute scars can be caused in the vaginal lining – not the tears that are sometimes made by rape, but little abrasions which can still be painful and slow to heal. But curiously, although lubrication may be impaired in an atrophic vagina which does not distend well, the situation is often improved if intercourse takes place regularly once or twice a week, which seems to restore some of the lost distensibility of the vagina. Unfortunately some women forgo intercourse because of anxiety or pain, and find the lubrication difficulty aggravated unless they use vaginal lubricants or are being treated with vaginal oestrogen; oestrogen by mouth may be required in addition.

Occasionally an older woman will experience acute abdominal pain during orgasm. This is another effect of pelvic shrinkage. Before the menopause the body of the uterus may be twice the size of the cervix, but with the general loss of oestrogen it may be reduced to half the size. Instead of contracting regularly and relaxing smoothly as it normally does at orgasm, the uterus in older women may go into spasm, which can be painful for a minute or two. This can often be avoided or relieved by treatment.

Like so many changes at the climacteric the impact of natural ageing becomes easily overlaid by psychological reactions and then psychosexual difficulties are encountered. They may be particularly disturbing for the woman who is marrying for the first time late in life, or has not had a sexual partner for many years and has previously relied for sexual relief on self-stimulation by one of the many methods of masturbation. Nothing destroys sexual effectiveness more at any age than personal doubts as to potential responsiveness. The great thing is to avoid recriminations. There are times when a man can't put on a good performance. He is annoyed with himself, and so gets angry with the woman. She is apt in turn to resent his 'failure'. Many psychosexual problems need never arise if men and women understand the genital changes which can be expected in the other as the years go by. These normal changes can be precipitated into abnormality by misconceptions fostered over generations. There should be no reason for a healthy man to suffer from the 'postmature' ejaculation problem or for the woman to retire into postmenopausal asexuality with its real danger of attendant marital discord.

# 6 The menopause and the skeleton

When I was a medical student we were taught – all too briefly, although our teachers didn't know any better – about a condition known in those days as 'menopausal osteoporosis', because it occurred in women, particularly if they had an early menopause. As you may have guessed, this phrase meant 'porous bones related to the menopause'. Today the condition is known simply as 'osteoporosis', because now we know that a minority of men get it too – though later in life and less severely than women, nature being, in the words immortalized by John Studd, 'a rotten gynaecologist, who doesn't look after women's ovaries, but only makes holes in her and in her bones'. About a quarter of all postmenopausal white women develop osteoporosis.

With increasing age both men and women suffer some loss of minerals, particularly calcium, from their bones. In men this process begins around the age of 50, about ten years later than it does in women, in whom the early mineral loss may precede the menopause by a number of years. The condition usually progresses slowly and is seldom sufficiently advanced to show X-ray changes within ten years of the natural menopause, though they may be evident within two years after a surgical menopause.

It has been estimated that after the age of 50, women lose 1% of the calcium from their bones each year; by the age of 70 approximately 15% and perhaps as much as 30% of the skeleton has been destroyed. Black people have denser bones to start with and their loss of bone is less noticeable. As calcium disappears from the skeleton it leaves enlarged spaces within the bone structure, which becomes spongy in appearance. Instead of new bone being laid down, more is resorbed. The porousness of the bones makes them brittle, and so more liable to break. As a side effect of the large amounts of calcium passed out from the bones and excreted in the blood and then in the urine, the condition may lead to the formation of kidney and bladder stones.

Aches and pains, especially in the shoulders, are frequently experienced at the time of the climacteric, particularly low backache, or as it is often referred to, 'lumbago'. At least a quarter of menopausal women suffer from major orthopaedic or bone troubles, including fractures and painful joints and muscles. Early bone changes may begin about two years after the menopause, though sometimes earlier, and experts believe that at the age of 40, 5%, at 50, 15%, at 60, 30%, at 70, 65%, and at 80, 85% of women show some degree of osteoporosis.

I often think of the mother of one of my American friends who, over about 20 years gradually shrank in size before our eyes, rather like Alice in Wonderland. As I went back to America every few years, I noticed she was smaller and shorter. Slowly her chin dropped forward on to her chest as her slim figure collapsed, and the hump on her back grew larger. She was seldom free from pain and relied, eventually, entirely on her intelligent and devoted husband for continuous care, because in the end she could not get out of her chair without help. It saddens me now to realize, in retrospect, what I did not understand in those days, that oestrogen, if given in time, probably could have halted the inexorable advancement of her osteoporosis, although it might not have been able to replace bone lost already. Another sad feature is that immobility adds to bone loss; women with osteoporosis should be as active as possible, although their pain often limits movement – as in the case of my friend's mother – and so a vicious circle is established.

Because osteoporosis is so much more common in women than in men after the age of 50, they are more subject to fractures of their bones than men, and this liability increases with age. By the time a woman is 50 a fracture of the hip at the neck of the femur or long thigh bone, where its head articulates as a ball-and-socket joint with the hip bone, is three times more likely to happen than to a man, four times more common at 60 and five times more common over the age of 70.

Such fractures of the hip requiring long immobilization in bed formerly killed one out of every three women who were unlucky enough to sustain them in a fall, and who often developed pneumonia and chest complications or bloodclots in their legs during the slow union of bones over a number of weeks, perhaps months. Now that active orthopaedic surgery enables the two broken ends of the bone to be aligned and held in position by a thick metal pin, which is later removed, the individual can get about, and the outlook is much better. But a fractured hip can still be grossly disabling, and other fractures can be a source of considerable incapacity.

Bone fractures due to osteoporosis are likely to happen after a trivial or apparently negligible injury: the latter may even pass unnoticed, and can be the result of stooping to open a drawer, pulling a bed out from a wall, leaning over to reach something, or even turning over in bed, as well, of course, as knocking an arm against a wall, tripping on a step, or merely being jostled in a supermarket.

The commonest sites of these osteoporotic fractures are the wrist and the hip. Fractures of the shoulder, spine and the arm also occur. Spinal fractures are troublesome, to say the least, and, unlike fractures which are caused by sudden serious injuries and falls in younger people, often progress insidiously. Spinal bones (vertebrae) if osteoporotic are liable to collapse on one another, resulting in the so-called 'crush' fractures which can contribute to the loss in height of up to as much as 18 centimetres. Women with crush fractures lose bone much more rapidly than other women. We are all familiar with the stooping figures of old ladies like my friend's mother, with humped backs, who are sometimes politely described as possessing the 'dowager's hump'. With 2.5 or 4 centimetres in variability, height and arm span measure the same, and excess of arm span is an indication of height loss. Arms do not get shorter because, unlike the spine, they do not have to bear weight. In women whose ovaries have been removed under the age of 45 it is common to find that their arm span is greater than their height, unless they have been treated wih oestrogen.

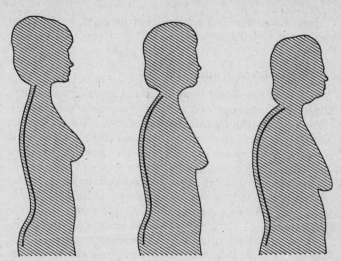

Progressive curvature of the spine

## Diagnosis

The density of bone can be measured by various advanced X-ray techniques. X-rays of the bones of the hand or forearm are usually used to estimate the degree of general bone loss as they reflect general changes elsewhere in the rest of the skeleton. The diagnosis of osteoporosis also rests on knowing the amounts of calcium and phosphorus excreted by the body. As these minerals are withdrawn from bone, higher than normal amounts of calcium and phosphorus are present in the blood and in the urine, and can be measured. Raised values of the amino-acid hydroxyproline in the blood and urine also indicate the amount of bone ground substance, apart from calcium, which is being lost. Such diagnostic tests are useful in confirming the onset of osteoporosis, in combination with X-rays, but some evidence is conflicting. For one thing the values for calcium and phosphorus in blood and urine can also be raised following the removal of the ovaries, though not after hysterectomy, unless the ovaries have been damaged in some way during the operation.

## Factors which affect osteoporosis

If calcium is withheld from the diet of experimental animals they develop osteoporosis. For no known reason the body prefers to sacrifice the skeleton than to allow the levels of calcium in the blood to fall. Certain factors concerned with the metabolism of calcium and phosphorus, which also play a part in the development of osteoporosis, affect the density of bone, among them Vitamin D, which helps to absorb calcium from the diet and deposits it in bone. Kidney function can influence the excretion of calcium and the intestinal function affects how much the body takes in. In addition, the hormones secreted by the thyroid and parathyroid glands exert a profound influence on bone formation, the parathyroid regulating the amount of calcium in the blood. Intestinal conditions which may prevent absorption of food may adversely affect the amount of calcium and Vitamin D available from the diet. And lastly there are sex steroids, the principal culprit being (how did you guess?) lack of oestrogen. Androgens or male hormones tend to promote osteoporosis in women, oestrogens to protect against its development.

## The role of oestrogen

Women who have osteoporosis often have other evidence of oestrogen deficiency, such as atrophic vaginitis, and often absorb calcium poorly from the food they eat. How does oestrogen – or rather its lack – manage to exert these far-reaching effects? Some of the answers lie in the probability that lack of oestrogen alters the response of bone to the actions of the parathyroid hormone and possibly the growth hormone too. The relevant action may take place at the nerve endings in the bones. As a result, the availability of calcium can be reduced in the absence of enough oestrogen to influence the hormonal action of the thyroid and increase the activity of the parathyroid with its regulatory effect on blood calcium. Secondly, oestrogen improves the absorptive power of the intestine, helping to promote absorption of calcium and so prevent deficiency in the body. It has also been suggested that in the absence of sufficient oestrogen the body cannot adapt to a diet low in calcium.

The relationship between osteoporosis and oestrogen deficiency was demonstrated over thirty-five years ago in young women who had developed an artificial menopause after surgical removal of the ovaries which promotes loss of bone comparable with that lost after a natural menopause. Removal of ovaries was frequently performed in the past at the same time as hysterectomy, the object usually being that, as the abdomen was already open at the operation to remove the uterus, the ovaries might as well be taken out for good measure, rather as surgeons now tend to take out the appendix; it was argued that this would eliminate any chance of their subsequently becoming malignant. In some cases they were, of course, already diseased or there was a definite indication for their removal. Today every effort is made by surgeons to conserve the ovaries of premenopausal women in order to avoid the subsequent development of osteoporosis and other oestrogen deficiencies. Surgeons also now realize how very seldom malignant changes arise in conserved ovaries; it has been calculated that the odds are a thousand to one against a woman of 45 having an ovarian cancer during her remaining lifespan.

**Medical research**

We owe a debt to the many women whose ovaries have been removed and whose misfortune has contributed to our knowledge of the effects of deprivation of oestrogen. Their experience and their cooperation in medical research has given us information which could not be obtained in other ways, and has taught us about the manifestations of true ovarian deficiency as in osteoporosis, and the effect of possible and suitable methods of its replacement. This has thrown further light on the disorders encountered at the natural menopause and has led to developments in their treatment. There may be some doubts as to the amount of oestrogen produced by the ovaries at a particular moment in the natural climacteric, but none after a surgical menopause, whose date can be accurately pinpointed, and this provides a base-line for evaluation of progress and treatment.

## Prevention

Valuable information on the development of osteoporosis was obtained by research on women without ovaries by Dr J. M. Aitken and his colleagues at the Western Infirmary, Glasgow between 1968 and 1971. Their research proved that osteoporosis does not develop when the ovaries are removed in women after the age of 45, even if they are still having periods at the time, and could therefore be assumed to be producing ovarian oestrogen until then. Before the age of 45 removal of the ovaries causes bone loss in osteoporosis which is directly related to the length of time the body was deprived of ovarian hormones; but after 45 the influence of the ovaries becomes less important, although they still make some precursors, and provide a little oestrogen.

Dr Aitken also investigated a number of Glasgow women whose ovaries had been removed two months, three years, and six years previously. He gave half of them oestrogen and the other half a placebo, and measured the density of their bones yearly. All the placebo-treated women continued to lose bone mass. Those who had been given oestrogen within two months of the removal of their ovaries lost no bone. In those treated within three years the bone mass increased, but in women who were not treated until six years after their operation, bone was lost in amounts equal to that lost by women who had been given only a placebo.

So it would appear likely that oestrogen loses its effect on bone by the time six years have elapsed after the menopause, though resorption can be prevented from developing if oestrogen is given within three years; this may even lead at this early stage to some restoration of lost bone. Recent research suggests that the addition of a progestogen in treatment further delays loss of bone, and may indeed lead to some replacement.

As the ovaries exert this protective effect, clearly the sooner the diagnosis of osteoporosis is made by the appropriate methods, the sooner treatment can be instigated, and the better chance there is of halting the process. The response to oestrogen treatment varies directly with the duration of oestrogen deprivation and with the dose of oestrogen which is given. In San Francisco Dr G. S. Gordan reduced the fracture rate in postmenopausal women by giving them oestrogen, and found the larger 1.25 mg dose of conjugated oestrogen more effective than the 0.625 mg dose.

During Dr Aitken's tests a curious seasonal variation in bone mass was discovered in women who were receiving the placebo. Their bone mass decreased between the summer and the winter, and increased in the spring. At the same time their urinary calcium and phosphate values fell in the spring, only to rise again in the autumn, parallel with the loss of bone. It seems likely that postmenopausal women may become more sensitive to the lack of Vitamin D – formed by the action of sunlight on the skin – in the sunless winter months. Possibly oestrogen abolishes this phenomenon, because it was not noticed in the oestrogen-treated group of women – with one interesting exception. In the spring of January to March 1971 a postal strike interrupted the supplies posted from the hospital to patients taking part in the oestrogen trial. This withdrawal of oestrogen was reflected in the biochemical analyses and in bone density which was temporarily diminished.

In Leeds Professor B. E. C. Nordin and his colleagues have confirmed a rapid bone loss in the five to ten years following the menopause, and believe that only oestrogen will retard this. At a later period malabsorption of calcium due to deficiency of Vitamin D may be improved by taking extra calcium as well as oestrogen. Some other studies have, it is true, produced conflicting reports on the role of calcium. We do not know if women who walk several miles a day get less osteoporosis than more sedentary women. Other questions remain unanswered, including why childless women and those of slim build are said – though this has not been substantiated – to be more prone to develop osteoporosis than fatter women who have had children. Nor is it clear why a woman may notice improvement in her aches and bone pains within two weeks of receiving oestrogen treatment, before any substantial bone changes could have taken place.

The aches and pains of which so many menopausal women complain may well be due to pressure on the nerves where they emerge from the spine in the region of collapsed vertebrae. But pain may also result from softening of ligaments and lack of strength in muscles. We know that the pelvic ligaments are affected by lack of oestrogen and lose their elasticity at the climacteric. The same failure to support bones may arise in relation to the spine and the rest of the skeleton.

Lactic acid builds up in the muscles after exercise, and its accumulation in muscles makes them ache until the lactic acid is dispersed. Oestrogen may promote the dispersal of lactic acid from muscles, and could be expected to restore some integrity of ligaments.

The disabling and crippling effect of osteoporosis is one of the most convincing arguments in favour of giving oestrogen on a long-term basis as a preventive to young women whose ovaries have been removed – provided the reason for their removal is known, and a progestogen is also given.

### Arthritic changes

Other bony disease must always be excluded. Many arthritic aches and pains of later life are degenerative in origin; the symptoms are not caused by lack of oestrogen nor improved by its administration. Certain conditions produce X-ray bone changes which closely mimic those found in osteoporosis; these are common at the age of the menopause, and recourse to other investigations may be necessary. It may be helpful to differentiate the pain of osteoporosis from that experienced in other conditions. Osteoporotic backache is often localized to the lower part of the spine or the middle of the back where bending is greatest. There may be tenderness at the site of a recent fracture, but the osteoporotic back pain tends to be generalized and does not characteristically radiate down the leg or arm as it may when arthritic bone changes in the spine constrict the nerves where they emerge.

## Prophylaxis

No one can put bone back after osteoporosis has occurred. We can only prevent more calcium being lost. As osteoporosis arises so frequently, so insidiously, so imperceptibly, and responds so well to early treatment and so poorly to late treatment, is there a case for every postmenopausal woman taking oestrogen to prevent osteoporosis developing? Even if the Health Service could afford this, which it could not, the consensus of medical opinion appears to be as given by Professor Sir John Dewhurst when president of the Royal College of Obstetricians and Gynaecologists (*The Menopause* 1976, edited by R. J. Beard).

'It is in this area of prevention of osteoporotic changes that the case for long-term prophylactic oestrogen therapy seems to me strongest. Its weakness is in our lack of knowledge about the frequency and degree of such changes if prophylaxis is not employed . . . I am obliged to conclude that at present we do not know the amount of symptomatic osteoporosis in the postmenopausal population, nor the extent to which this is concerned with oestrogen deprivation as distinct from ageing alone.'

Sir John Dewhurst's argument rests on the belief that because of the many factors involved in the development of osteoporosis the cessation of ovarian function may be the trigger, rather than the main cause. The same difficulty crops up here, as with other conditions at the climacteric, in separating the effects of ageing from those of added deficiency of oestrogen. Osteoporosis cannot be a straight deficiency disease, but is rather a manifestation of other defects. Oestrogen can only halt or slow the process. A diet containing adequate amounts of protein, calcium and Vitamin D may help, as do general measures aimed at keeping as mobile as possible. To give oestrogen for life to women to prevent osteoporosis developing after the menopause may theoretically be a good idea, if expensive. Large doses would probably be needed and treatment initiated early. Until more is known of the hazards this is not justifiable, or even practical, and would entail very close and frequent supervision of every woman so treated. But it would certainly reduce the cost of treating the many older women with fractures who occupy hospital beds and attend our orthopaedic out-patient departments.

# 7 The climacteric and the heart and the blood vessels

Men have an advantage over women where osteoporosis is concerned; the balance is partially redressed for women in the case of diseases of the heart and blood vessels – until they reach the age at which the menopause occurs. Until this period is reached, men are at much greater risk of dying of coronary artery disease. After the menopause women, who have until then enjoyed relative immunity to today's major killer gradually revert to parity with men. 28% of all women in the UK who die between the ages of 45 and 54 do so from coronary heart disease. For men in the same age groups the figure soars to over 50%. At 44 a woman is fourteen or fifteen times less likely to develop coronary artery disease than a man, but by the time she is 70 the risks are nearly equal. In both sexes coronary artery disease increases sharply in middle life and continues thereafter, but men are handicapped by ten to fifteen years. For them the rise usually begins earlier than in women, when they are in their early forties, and sometimes even sooner.

It would be logical to attribute the relative protection against heart disease in younger women to the effect of oestrogen, and to postulate that its withdrawal at the menopause causes the increased vulnerability. But the male advantage is not constant in all societies. It is, for example, virtually absent in the American negro in the southern states, in the Japanese, who have very little coronary disease, and in the Bantu, where nutritional and economic factors may operate. The 'protection' is more likely to be associated with other factors in which hormones may play a related part. Doctors at St Mary's Hospital, London have suggested recently that in fact it may not be a question of women losing protection, but of men losing their vulnerability after 50, when *their* supplies of testosterone fall significantly.

In the last twenty years the increasing volume of coronary artery disease has taken on epidemic proportions in Western society, although it is no longer rising in the United States. In Britain the rise in the death rate has been steeper in women than in men. Between 1958 and 1972 it increased by 50% in women aged 35 to 44, and by 36% in those aged 45 to 54. The increase has been negligible in women who are aged 55 to 64. However, there has not been a proportionate increase from one age group to the next, and no acceleration in the death rate in the menopausal years. It is unlikely, therefore, that the menopause alone increases women's liability to coronary heart disease.

The reason why younger women have become more vulnerable is not clear, but let us look at the way clotting or thrombosis occurs in arteries and veins and at the factors which increase the risk of coronary artery disease developing.

## Coronary artery disease

The coronary arteries, as part of the general circulation, supply the heart muscle (myocardium) with its blood. The big coronary arteries lie on the surface of the heart, and the smaller ones penetrate the myocardium; they carry nourishment, and small capillaries link the little arteries with veins which in turn take the used blood back into larger veins.

Like other arteries in the body the coronaries degenerate with age, but the effect is greater in them than in other arteries. Fatty streaks appear in the lining of arteries, sometimes quite early in life; as these increase with time they may enlarge to form plaques in the arterial wall on which blood products including the small bodies known as platelets settle, forming a deposit in which the fatty substance cholesterol and calcium accumulate. The plaques get increasingly harder, and the whole wall of the artery may eventually become scarred and more rigid as the plaques get bigger. The resulting condition is known as atherosclerosis or hardening of the arteries. Coronary atherosclerosis may progress to obstruction of the blood flow as the calcified or atheromatous deposits narrow, and may eventually close the artery completely. This slow process develops over a number of years. X-rays have shown that by the age of 50 to 60 there are deposits of calcium in the aorta, the main artery of the body, in 25% of men, and 13% of women. After 60, women overtake men, and deposit more calcium in the walls of their arteries as they lose calcium from the bones. The pain in the chest which is experienced in coronary artery disease is referred to as angina; it usually comes on with exertion because the heart is then required to pump more blood round its narrowed, calcified, and, therefore, less-efficient arteries.

Clots of blood are liable to form on an area in a blood vessel which is already damaged. In the brain, the result may be a stroke. In a coronary artery if a large clot (thrombus) forms on top of an atheromatous calcified plaque it cuts off more of the blood supply to the heart muscle, the process being known as 'infarction', and the area deprived of blood a 'myocardial infarct', which is the usual sequence of coronary thrombosis.

Clotting in an artery, as in coronary thrombosis, must not be confused with venous thrombosis, or clotting in a vein, where the damage is not necessarily incurred at the site of the thrombus. Here the danger is that the clot may detach itself and be carried round the body as an embolus in the main bloodstream and lodge in another blood vessel. Thrombo-embolism can cause a stroke if a clot blocks a blood vessel in the brain. Alternatively a thrombus may block one of the veins carrying blood to the lungs – a process known as pulmonary embolism. In either instance the severity of the effect depends on the size and position of the clot. A large one may cause sudden heart failure and death, and in the brain, paralysis. Small clots may cause trivial effects, and even pass unnoticed.

### Risk factors

In men three major factors are associated with coronary artery disease. They are *raised lipids*, the fatty substance bound to proteins in the blood, *cigarette smoking*, particularly if heavy, and *high blood pressure*. The same risk factors are prominent in women who develop coronary artery disease under the age of 45.

*Raised lipids.* The influence of animal fats in the diet in promoting the development of atherosclerosis is still the subject of unresolved conflicting medical opinion, but a relationship between the blood lipids or fats and cardiovascular disease is now accepted. The principal fats are cholesterol, triglycerides and lipoproteins. In the condition known as familial hyperlipidaemia, an inherited tendency, the blood fats are unduly high even in the first year of life. Normally they rise steadily throughout adult life, the increase beginning around 15, though the effect on the arteries may not be seen for thirty or thirty-five years. Although the total lipids rise with age irrespective of sex – by as much as 30% in some instances – there are differences in the amount and composition or proportion of blood lipids in men and premenopausal women. These differences disappear after the menopause, the time when women are more prone to develop coronary artery disease.

If the ovaries are removed before the age of 40 the total blood lipids increase, the rise being higher when both are removed than when only one ovary is taken away, another factor predisposing to coronary heart disease. The hormonal effect on cholesterol is evident during the menstrual cycle, when the amount varies, dropping by as much as 15% at ovulation, when oestrogen levels are at their highest. After the menopause lipoproteins, triglycerides and cholesterol all rise by up to 20% of their premenopausal level. Lipids are also significantly higher in women who have a menopause before they are 40 than in women who stop menstruating later, the rise being proportional to the woman's age at the premature menopause.

While oestrogen lowers the amount of cholesterol in the blood – though this has been contested in one recent study of treatment – at the same time it induces a significant rise in the triglycerides in the blood. In this way oestrogen may contribute to clot formation in which triglycerides play an important part. It does not provide the protection against the development of atherosclerosis, as might be expected, but could possibly accelerate its development by increasing clot-promoting triglycerides. Although it may lower one factor, cholesterol, the triglycerides rise counteracts this effect. Treatment with oestrogen for cancer of the prostate in men caused more men to die from heart conditions than could be expected to die in the three months following the operation. Treatment with oestrogen of postmenopausal women who had had myocardial infarction has had a similar deleterious effect. Paradoxically, although oestrogen might seem to protect women before the menopause from the coronary artery disease to which men are so much more prone, giving oestrogen to postmenopausal women, although their own stocks are then low, may possibly increase the risk instead of preventing coronary artery disease.

Blood clots in a few minutes when it escapes from an artery or from a vein, as part of nature's protective action to heal the breach. There are two mechanisms here. One depends on the presence in the blood itself of special clotting enzymes known loosely as 'clotting factors'. The second mechanism involves changes at the site of breach or injury in the artery or the vein. The platelets become more liable to stick to one another and to the injured area over which fibrin, a blood protein, is deposited. Oestrogens influence some of the clotting factors, affect fibrin formation and increase the adhesiveness and aggregation of platelets. Laboratory studies have shown that clotting takes place more quickly in the presence of oestrogen, particularly, though not only, the synthetic oestrogens, but this depends more on the dose than the type of oestrogen given.

*Cigarette smoking.* Parallel with the rise in coronary artery disease in the past twenty years cigarette smoking has also increased, especially among women. Between 1958 and 1970 the average consumption of cigarettes smoked by women in the UK increased by 35% and doubled in women aged 16 to 25 years. Studies in Ireland, Sweden, Scotland and England have shown that more women smokers have heart attacks than women who do not smoke. There is no evidence that such women's smoking was in any way related to the menopause, and it is generally accepted that the increase in earlier smoking is likely to have contributed to the rise in female coronary artery disease, there being no doubt of the strong link between smoking and coronary thrombosis.

*High blood pressure.* The blood pressure increases in both men and women as we get older, but the menopause itself has no direct effect on it. However, oestrogens may cause a rise in blood pressure in susceptible women. Young women whose blood pressure is already high do not have the same immunity to cardiovascular disease as other women, and are liable to develop coronary heart disease just as early as men. This may be why there is no sex difference in the age of onset of coronary artery disease in American negroes who live in the southern states where raised blood pressure is relatively common in women.

## Venous thrombosis

Apart from the recent increase in the number of deaths from coronary artery disease in women, the increased use of the contraceptive pill has affected venous thrombosis, or clotting in veins. The controlled retrospective studies carried out in the United Kingdom by Vessey and Doll, and in the United States, and the prospective study by the Royal College of General Practitioners, reported in 1974, have all established that during the reproductive years of a woman's life oral contraceptives increase the likelihood of her developing deep vein thrombosis and pulmonary embolism at least five times. Some research workers think that the synthetic oestrogens used in the Pill may promote clotting more readily than the natural oestrogens used for hormone treatment at the climacteric, but others believe this is not so with the very small doses of synthetic oestrogens which can be used to treat menopausal symptoms. There is laboratory evidence that an increase in some – though not all – of the clotting factors in the blood can occur in women after only three months' treatment with natural oestrogens, the changes being reversed when oestrogen treatment is stopped. When oestrogen was given to men with cardiovascular disease *both* natural and synthetic oestrogens appeared to increase venous thrombosis.

But while one in every two thousand women a year who take the Pill develops a clot in the veins, usually the deep leg veins, there have been so few studies in menopausal women under treatment that the relationship of venous thrombosis, if any, to the effect of oestrogen is not known. For this we shall have to wait for the results of research which is now being done in America, where the large numbers of women taking oestrogen provide researchers with more material than is available in Britain.

## Artificial and premature menopause: its effect on the heart and blood vessels

Although coronary heart disease is still uncommon in young and middle-aged women, those who have an early menopause are more likely to develop it than women whose menopause occurs later. A small study in Edinburgh in 1963 indicated that women whose menopause occurred before they were 40, when followed up by Professor Michael Oliver after ten to twenty years, had developed seven times as much coronary artery disease as a comparable group of healthy women in an Edinburgh general practice.

In Sweden another study in menopausal women who had had myocardial infarction showed that 76% of these women compared with another 48% of healthy control women had had the menopause before they were 50, although there is no evidence to prove that oestrogen would have prevented the infarction.

Removing the ovaries under the age of 40 can have a similar effect on the subsequent development of vascular heart disease. In 1963 a group of American doctors found that women who had their ovaries removed before they were 40 were nearly five times more likely than other women to develop disease of the heart or its blood vessels. The investigators compared the records of two sets of women; 102 had had their ovaries removed and 112 had had a simple hysterectomy without removal of ovaries. In the latter group 4 women developed angina and 3 had signs of myocardial disease. Among the women whose ovaries had been removed, 15 developed angina and 19 showed signs of myocardial disease. By examining hospital records the same investigators further proved that there was a significant difference between young women without ovaries who had been treated with oestrogen, and those who had not, cardiovascular disease being significantly higher in the untreated group.

Although some reports in this field are conflicting, the high rate of coronary heart disease in women whose ovaries have been removed and the rise to parity with men of women after the menopause is not in dispute, only its mechanism. From the available evidence it is clear that oestrogen does not protect the menopausal woman from the rise in blood lipids which is associated with increased cardiovascular disease.

## The future

A recent American study has failed to find a statistically significant relationship between taking oestrogen and developing postmenopausal myocardial infarction, but the numbers of women who had taken oestrogen were relatively small. It has, however, been suggested more than once that we may find thrombo-embolism occurring more frequently, and possibly an increase in coronary artery disease which takes longer to develop, as hormone treatment is extended. Women who are likely to be most at risk of developing coronary artery disease are heavy smokers, women in whose family other members have suffered from coronary artery disease and those who have high blood lipids and high blood pressure. Women who fall into one or other category, particularly the smokers and those with a family history of coronary artery disease, may be considered to be unsuited for oestrogen treatment.

It becomes increasingly important to find which formulations and doses of oestrogen will relieve menopausal distress without accelerating the bloodclotting mechanisms. By the time they reach the normal menopause women are already predisposed to an enhancement of clotting because some of the clotting factors alter with age, and, in addition, the blood begins to flow more sluggishly in the smaller peripheral arteries and veins in older people. Their circulation is not as good and this makes clotting more likely. Many doctors think that the danger of precipitation of clotting disorders at the menopause if oestrogen is given is at least as great as the danger of causing endometrial cancer which has received so much more attention.

There is, however, no clinical evidence so far that giving oestrogen for the climacteric syndrome has as yet significantly increased the amount of venous or arterial thrombosis when used in acceptable doses, but some cardiologists see the possibility that this may show up.

It must be remembered that the oestrogens in the Pill are given to younger women, and in much larger doses and in a different form from the smaller doses of oestrogen given to women at the menopause; the latter may be as low as the equivalent of one third of the oestrogen in even a low-oestrogen Pill. And Professor Martin Vessey, whose extensive epidemiological work on the Pill at Oxford enables him to speak with authority, says: 'Giving the Pill to young women and giving oestrogen to menopausal women are completely different situations, and there is every reason to believe that the effects will be totally different. It is well established that there is a relationship between venous thrombosis, stroke and coronary thrombosis in young women and oral contraceptives. Whether there is a similar relationship in older women and oestrogens as hormone treatment remains to be seen.'

The main reason for caution is that the older woman is already at greater risk of a clotting disorder.

# 8 The management of the climacteric and its treatment

Treatment for menopausal problems is not simply a matter of getting a doctor to prescribe hormones, useful as they may be. It may often be a question of managing the situation, bearing in mind the effect of the personality of the woman and her circumstances. Some women remain unscathed by the menopause, some manage to overcome the problems themselves. Others need help.

The degree to which women need medical help is usually conditioned by their personality. Particularly vulnerable women are those who over the years have regarded their femininity in terms of their bodily functions. Menstruation, pregnancy and motherhood give the body its feminine significance. To women who see themselves bereft of their femininity in the ending of these functions the menopause comes as a partial death, with many attendant depressive and other symptoms. Remember Elizabeth of Chapter 2?

The type of woman who is unmoved by the menopause sees it impersonally and accepts it unquestioningly as being part of life. The days of such women have usually been filled with their homes, their job, caring for children and grandchildren. Their lives have not varied greatly since marriage. Sex plays no great part in it and sexual intercourse is regarded more as a duty than anything else. They are not the ones who seek much medical treatment and would not want it except in an emergency. Their expectations of life are based on its continuation within pre-existing conditions. The menopause may even be seen as a blessing because the periods and pregnancy interfere with the work pattern. As a rule such women neither expect, nor often need, help. Another type of woman, with an equally, if not more supportive, background in a secure family and social life, accepts that the menopausal years bring troubles, but she can cope with them. Ageing is not usually a threat, but if it turns out to be so such women do not look on it in a pessimistic way. Their home, hobbies, work or religion give them a purpose in life.

Lastly, there is a type of more dynamic woman who takes the menopause more aggressively, and may think her menopausal friends too soft. Because she has always managed to handle a situation and avert a crisis she looks first for ways of helping herself. Only when this fails does she take advantage of medical help.

There is of course no doubt that self-help often works and here are a few guidelines to be going on with.

## Self-help

The International Health Foundation showed in its report *The Menopause* that about a fifth of menopausal women find life becomes less interesting at the time of the climacteric, particularly after the menopause. One third of the women interviewed had jobs outside their homes, and these women were much more likely to disagree with the idea that the menopause made life more boring.

Boredom encourages introspection. In order to avoid dwelling on personal troubles it may be a good idea to move on to a more disciplined track than to sit at home gazing into the fire or languishing in the garden. A woman could, with advantage, then take on some regular commitment, or a job, and not mind too much if it is not paid as well as her experience, training or present skill lead her to think she merits. There may be compensations. In addition to being less bored herself she may also become less boring to others. No one likes a moaner, and a long-suffering saint can also irritate.

It is important not to let the appearance deteriorate, especially as the idea of the menopause is usually associated with distaste for, and even dread of, ageing. If a woman looks good she will like herself better, and so will everyone else. So any menopausal woman might with advantage give her wardrobe an overhaul, and pay more attention to hair, hands and feet. The middle-age spread is unflattering and uncomfortable. It is important to keep down weight and if seriously overweight to reduce it. Alcohol has a lot of calories, is a depressant, and large doses are best avoided. Lay off between-meal snacks.

With regard to personal relationships, especially those within the family circle, and of course at work, it is useful to remember that some element of psychiatric disturbance, usually transitory, is not uncommon at the climacteric. Having accepted this possibility, family and friends should be persuaded to do the same. Both sides will require a degree of tolerance and an understanding of the other's troubles. Make allowances for them as well as for yourself. But do not set too high a standard. Human nature is frail. You can comfort yourself that, although you feel tired and confused, depressed, and unable to make decisions now, nothing lasts for ever, not even the climacteric.

Insomnia is likely to be one of your troubles, but at the same time you don't want to get up in the morning and prefer to sleep in the daytime. One way to avoid this is to make sure you are physically exhausted by bedtime. Exercise during the day will help your weight problem and improve your general health. An evening walk should ensure a greater degree of tiredness and a more relaxed attitude towards the coming night and so improve your chances of sleeping well.

Then you could try the proverbial hot drink at bedtime, or even a nightcap. Many a good nurse has proved that tepid sponging, fresh pillows, a newly-made bed and a drink, work as well as a sleeping pill, though you may sometimes find you need a sleeping pill or soporific as well.

And on the subject of drinks: beware of endless cups of coffee during the day or too many cups of tea last thing at night. The caffeine in coffee is a stimulant and increases the awareness of pain. And hot drinks can make flushes and sweats more uncomfortable. Tea also contains caffeine, and tends to increase the flow of urine. If you drink a lot of fluid before you go to bed you may find you have to get up more often to pass water.

Flushes and sweats are precipitated by stress and excitement. Although it is easier said than done, there is no harm in trying to avoid this.

Lastly, if the vagina is dry and intercourse is uncomfortable, it will be improved if you use a lubricant such as KY jelly or a vaginal cream or jelly of the contraceptive variety. It is important not to stop having regular sexual intercourse, or marital and psychological problems may build up. These can be very upsetting and may become insoluble if allowed to develop for too long. Sex is relaxing and makes you feel young and happy – why throw away one of life's major pleasures, when by sharing it you can make someone else happy too?

## Medical help

Once you have decided that you want to consult a doctor you are ill-advised to by-pass your general practitioner. He or she should already know more about you, your medical history and your circumstances than others who know you less well. *Moreover it is essential to see him/her if you have any bleeding between the periods, if you have a bloody discharge, irregular bleeding or excessive flooding.* Conditions which are unrelated to the menopause, and possibly serious, may arise at this time of life. Correct diagnosis, both of the latter possible states and of true oestrogen deficiency, is essential before beginning treatment. There may be personal and individual contra-indications to treatment which the general practitioner will want to consider.

Although television programmes have had great influence in informing women about the menopause, the majority of women appear to have derived much of their knowledge about the menopause from magazines. We owe a great debt to the women who have written and canvassed so energetically to bring the needs of women and the help that is available not only into public but also into medical consciousness. Nevertheless, while much important information has been relayed, some bad reporting has also occurred. Although journalists have helped numerous women, a few have succeeded in confusing and even in antagonizing a minority of doctors. So use your common sense when you get to the surgery.

A surprising number of men evidently read women's magazines, and the lady who comes to see her general practitioner waving a glossy in one hand, and opens the conversation with the words 'My husband says I need it' ('it' being oestrogen) may get a cool reception. It is difficult for a doctor to take kindly to a verbose patient, or to one who cannot describe her symptoms clearly without too much emotion, or say when they first became noticeable.

It would be a good thing to have kept a note of the numbers of hot flushes experienced each day and at night. Records of dates of periods or any irregular bleeding are important, and it would be useful to be able to describe any changes in the menstrual flow, its amount, colour and duration.


## Misconceptions

Hormone treatment has been used much more extensively and for a longer time in America than in Britain, and American women who pay for their drugs expect to get medical prescriptions when they want them. They have been heard in Britain to complain that doctors are conservative and resistant to the idea that women who want oestrogen should be given it on demand. Some have British friends to whom they have passed on the idea that oestrogen provides the answer to the secret of perpetual youth. While many women undoubtedly suffer from very distressing symptoms which oestrogen relieves, others sometimes expect the same treatment to be successful in relieving minor symptoms which may not even be related to the menopause. Do not expect your doctor to prescribe oestrogen as a rejuvenator, although it does seem to improve the condition of the hair and skin, and can in this sense be rejuvenating.

Misconceptions have arisen because women have found that oestrogen is a mental tonic, and, as already described, generally cheers them up and helps them to cope with worries or problems. But many symptoms which seem to be relieved by taking oestrogen are not specifically caused by its deficiency.

## Domino effect

Oestrogen, as I have said, almost invariably immediately improves flushing and sweating. Because flushing and sweating cause discomfort and therefore insomnia, insomnia generates anxiety, and anxiety fatigue, fatigue contributes to inefficiency and confusion, and this to forgetfulness and irritability, and the lot to depression, women might be excused for thinking that all these secondary effects when experienced on their own are also curable by oestrogen. In fact, they improve when oestrogen improves the primary condition and are really cured by the 'domino' action already described.

A comparable sequence of events, though less spectacular, follows when oestrogen is given for vaginal dryness and soreness, and the allied changes in the urethra and bladder. As the atrophic vaginitis improves, psychosexual anxiety may become less. When sexual intercourse ceases to be painful or difficult, and therefore unwelcome, sexual desire or libido may improve, resulting in more harmonious sexual relations. Insomnia could be less of a nuisance as the sufferer ceases to get up so often in the night, perhaps waking her partner in the process, but the domino effect has been shown in studies by Professor Stuart Campbell and his colleagues at the Chelsea Hospital for Women in London to be less where atrophic vaginitis is concerned than when related to the relief from flushing.

Their particular study was designed to measure the psychological menopausal state and its response to treatment. But as so often happens, if you look for one thing you find another. In order to assess the effects of oestrogen, controlled trials were instigated in different groups of patients. Some patients, who did not know they were receiving an inert placebo and not oestrogen, reported an improvement in vasomotor symptoms, and others that their vaginal dryness had improved on the placebo. The domino effect was apparent when other symptoms, including insomnia, improved in the women whose flushes had improved on the placebo. Insomnia was *not* however improved with the reported amelioration of vaginal dryness by the women who were still taking only the placebo, although their memory was said to be better and their anxiety less. The domino effect was negligible here.

## Medical attitudes to the climacteric

Although oestrogens have been used for many years in England to help to relieve distressing menopausal symptoms, especially after premature or surgical menopause, British doctors have undeniably been, and many still are, slow to accept the wider use of hormone treatment at the climacteric. If they thought about it at all, the last generation of doctors was likely to regard the menopause as something women had to get on with. In their turn women have been, though perhaps understandably – at least earlier on – unduly reticent about discussing their marital and intimate problems with men – and there are more men than women doctors. But both patients and doctors are far less inhibited today and able to speak more frankly to one another, though many women who could be helped still do not come forward. In a pilot study in 1976 in a practice of 40,000 patients 4.6% of women aged 40 to 49, and 5.9% aged 50 to 59 had received an oestrogen preparation, apart from the contraceptive pill, but nearer 15% to 20% of such women would probably benefit from hormone treatment.

There are still too many doctors who shy away from even considering the psychosexual problems of menopausal women. Either they are really oblivious to them, or expect they will go away on their own. Psychosexual problems can be very real and they *don't* always go away on their own. Fortunately these problems are becoming more widely recognized as an additional strain at the time of the climacteric. They may be precipitated by the climacteric itself or at least enhanced by it.

Some of the newer and more enthusiastic advocates of hormone treatment have been women doctors, especially those who have personal experience of the climacteric. One such convert says she could not understand why she had been feeling so strange recently, irritable, forgetful and confused. She suffered from the TATT (Tired All The Time) syndrome – was sometimes unable to remember the name of a certain shop, let alone who she had promised to go and see, and would forget the contents of a particular letter or where she had put her mail. The reason dawned on her one day, when she realized she was having a hot flush. She had never previously considered the possibility of being menopausal because her periods were only mildly irregular. The premenopausal women may often be in greater need of help than women who show overt signs of oesttrogen deficiency, and who can more easily recognize the climacteric state because the periods have ceased.

There has been an increasing acceptance of the value of hormone treatment by doctors whose attitudes have undoubtedly been swayed by the increasing popular demand consequent on the publicity in the lay press. In 1973/74 it was estimated by the pharmaceutical industry that some 50,000 UK women were receiving hormone treatment for the menopausal symptoms. In 1978 the figure was nearer 200,000. Market research by one major pharmaceutical company found that 48% of doctors approved of giving hormones for specific disorders. Those doctors who did not prescribe hormones gave as their reasons the risk of side effects, especially cancer, the risk of thrombosis, the possibility that the treatment might cause irregular menstrual bleeding, and either disapproved of interference with a 'natural process' or thought the efficacy and safety of the treatment had not yet been proved.

The investigators found that general practitioners were not always well informed about the climacteric and noticed great diversity of opinion among them. But over 80% were treating over half their menopausal patients with drugs unless the symptoms were mild or their patients responded to reassurance and explanation, or the patients were unwilling to accept the drugs. Rather more doctors prescribed hormones than those who prescribed sedatives, tranquillizers and antidepressant drugs for menopausal conditions. About 22% used hormones in three-quarters of their menopausal patients, and 42% in more than half their patients. The bulk of the treatment was given for flushes and sweats. Nine out of ten doctors expected that their patients' symptoms would last for more than a year and the majority considered that they would require treatment for over six months.

Another way of looking at the attitudes of the medical profession is to consider the actual number of prescriptions for menopausal treatment. The proportion which do not contain hormones is still quite high. On a recent estimate oestrogen products alone or in combination accounted for 55% and combinations of sex hormones for 12% of all prescriptions given for menopausal conditions. Of the rest, antispasmodics accounted for 10%, tranquillizers and sedatives for 9%, and other preparations such as pain relievers and a non-hormonal preparation, Dixarit, for 14%. Dixarit is intended to relieve migraine but may have some effect on the symptoms of oestrogen deficiency, although not an oestrogen-containing preparation.

In the UK there has been more than a three-fold increase in prescriptions for oestrogens other than oral contraceptives since the early seventies. This may be the result of the changing attitudes of doctors, but it has followed the journalistic crusade which alerted doctors to the needs of their patients. We may well ask whether doctors or their patients are responsible for the increased demand for hormonal pharmaceutical products.

## Specialist advice

The general practitioner is ideally the best person to look after menopausal conditions if they are straightforward. He has, as in all other conditions, access to consultants in case of need. But some practitioners do not as yet feel equipped for routine management of menopausal problems, and have neither the time nor the inclination to become closely involved. Others, we know, have been disturbed by conflicting reports, in both the lay and medical press, as to the safety of hormone treatment. We are far from knowing all there is to know about the climacteric, the reason why certain symptoms arise and the effects of long-term treatment. We do know that all medical care is a balancing of one risk against another. This requires experience and, in the case of hormone treatment, knowledge which was not available when many of today's doctors were students. Even today the subject is often dealt with briefly and inadequately in the crowded medical curriculum, and as yet there is not much postgraduate training in this field. Family doctors may reasonably argue that the menopause is not a killer – except of the quality of life – and this provides further reason for the exercise of caution, and, ultimately, perhaps, an excuse for shelving the responsibility for treatment. Specialist advice is available in hospitals, or more conveniently in one of the increasing number of menopause clinics, mainly attached to hospitals, which have been established in most big cities now. There the consultant will keep the general practitioner informed of the diagnosis, treatment and progress of all referred patients. (See page 149 for a list of menopause clinics.)

## Menopause clinics

An early menopause clinic in England – at the Birmingham Midland Hospital for Women – owed its formation in 1973 to a young gynaecologist, John Studd, who was impressed with the results of hormone treatment in America. Having notified the Birmingham doctors of the intention to start a menopause clinic and inviting them to refer patients, John Studd proceeded with three objectives in mind.

The first was to assess the need for a menopause clinic within a university department of Obstetrics and Gynaecology, as part of the National Health Service gynaecological care available to a community. Apart from the resulting medical observations, the number of similar clinics which have since been formed has given substantial evidence of their value and need and many now have a waiting list of at least three months. These clinics are filled with strikingly happy clients, in contrast, unfortunately, with some other out-patient departments.

The second objective was to evaluate the results of treatment, any side effects and the safety of differing regimes employed. Many women, once they have realized what hormones can do for them, insist that they don't care what the risks are and even go on to say they will gladly take a chance on a shorter happy life than a long gloomy one. Of course, another type of woman is more likely to be apprehensive. But whatever the views of their patients, doctors owe it to them to inform them to the best of their ability of all possible effects of treatment. Evaluation of this turns on research, which is most appropriately carried out in connection with a menopause clinic.

Lastly, besides the research aspect involved in the actual treatment of patients, it was hoped to elucidate with the help of laboratory assistance the biochemical and hormonal changes in the body at the time of the climacteric and their effects on the functioning of cells. Now menopause clinics aim to offer service-orientated research. No other source can provide the quantity or quality of research material by analysis of carefully kept records, complemented by laboratory investigations which are usually more conveniently carried out in a hospital laboratory. Some simpler tests can also be performed in an out-patient department catering for gynaecological patients.

Menopause clinics appeal to women because, perhaps for the first time, they are able to describe their problems to someone who is interested, and can get a sympathetic hearing from a doctor who has the time to listen. General practitioners may not have time for prolonged discussions, and outside a teaching hospital a gynaecologist may be allocated no more than ten minutes for each new patient. This enables him to make a general and a pelvic examination and a diagnosis, but not always to take a detailed, including a psychological, history.

In a menopause clinic it should be possible for gynaecologists to allow half to three-quarters of an hour for the first visit, perhaps even longer, and fifteen minutes for subsequent visits. At the initial visit, and subsequently as indicated, a full gynaecological examination is made, which usually includes cervical screening, a vaginal smear and examination of the urine. The blood pressure is also taken, and any other relevant examination is made, including examination of the breasts. Thereafter women are usually seen at first at three-monthly intervals, then six-monthly intervals, according to the progress made, and finally at longer intervals depending on the treatment. The general practitioner may be happy to take over the follow-up treatment, and arrange a fuller examination when this is indicated. This may include a suction curettage which is important because it monitors changes in the endometrium which may arise on treatment with oestrogen as a result of overstimulation.

## Menopause clinics as preventive medicine

The provision of continuing care and screening which women who attend a menopause clinic receive is one of the most important functions of the clinic, constituting as it does the best sort of preventive medicine like the 'well woman' clinics which are now popular. In the middle years a woman is increasingly prone to develop degenerative and possibly malignant disease. With the regular examinations that are made in a menopause clinic these conditions can be recognized early, perhaps before they have given rise to symptoms. At this stage they are, of course, more amenable to treatment. At the Birmingham clinic, in two years gynaecologists detected breast tumours in two women and a malignant skin tumour in another. One woman was found to have diabetes and three cervical smears showed a need for further investigation.

The early diagnosis of such illnesses reduces the longer-term demands on hospital beds and saves the Health Service considerable expenditure. Moreover, since the menopause disables women at a time when, if they are in jobs, they contribute substantially to the national economy, their disability can then be a load on the state. Yet menopause clinics are often largely dependent on help from pharmaceutical and other outside bodies for their research funds.

## Menopause clinics and the family doctor

There are now some forty menopause clinics both private and within National Health Service Hospitals which do valuable work in helping us to understand the problems of the climacteric (see page 149). Apart from the research aspect they also act as back-ups for doctors whose patients have specific problems, such as bleeding while on treatment, or who require additional investigation or supervision. But it would be a pity if the menopause clinic became in the public mind the only place where a woman could get treament for the climacteric syndrome. This lies most appropriately, as already stated, with the family doctor in the ordinary course of events. Specialist care is required for only a small minority of menopausal women. Most doctors will willingly give a woman the necessary letter for the nearest menopause clinic if they prefer not to treat a woman themselves.

## Counselling

It is logical to postulate that better socio-economic conditions make the climacteric less troublesome and easier to endure. Poverty and bad housing contribute to the difficulties encountered in middle age, though women who are less privileged may have less time to dwell on the problems of the climacteric. Those who live in a one-street village are more likely to think nothing can be done for the menopause. For them counselling is important. Better-educated women may need less counselling but tend to ask for it more frequently. Women who are not so well educated are often unwilling to ask for help, or may be unaware that the help is round the corner. Whoever a woman turns to at the climacteric, whether it is her general practitioner or the consultant to whom she has been referred, she will be helped in almost every instance by the ensuing discussion.

Explanations take time, but are the essence of good medical treatment. Fear, particularly in middle age, is often uppermost in many women's minds, particularly fear of malignant disease. This very fear is why some women delay asking for help. 'As long as it's not cancer,' they say when they finally appear at a menopause clinic, and obtain great relief when they can openly discuss their fears. It is particularly helpful for a woman to understand which of her symptoms are due to oestrogen deficiency and which to general wear and tear. She may then be able to adjust her mind to the fact that the end of youth which she has dreaded may not necessarily be a disaster. It is hardest for women who have grown up as beauties, and who have been preoccupied with their looks rather than their minds. Not so Elizabeth Taylor who is reported to have said: 'I love every one of my wrinkles' and has gone from strength to strength in spite of them. A woman doctor predicts that the menopause would probably distress Miss Taylor less than more fearful women.

Apart from the dread of cancer and of ageing there are women who want to be assured that they are not pregnant. Equally there are women, particularly those who are childless, who become obsessed with the wish for a child, and when hope finally disappears become very disturbed and may require specialist counselling.

The climacteric coincides with the time when marriages sustained for the sake of children who become independent about this time are already breaking down. While treatment for her climacteric symptoms may so improve her spirit that a wife is then able to summon up the will to end an unhappy marriage and make a successful new life, marriage guidance counselling can in some other circumstances salvage a less permanently damaged marriage which is heading for the rocks.

More serious psychological problems may call for the help of a psychiatrist and for psychotherapy. Both husband and wife may benefit from psychosexual counselling and re-education. Failure to stimulate the partner, persistent premature ejaculation on the man's part and inability to relax on the woman's part are the main factors which cause sexual activity to fail. These can be helped by the modern psychological techniques which are now available to couples who really wish to improve their sex life.

It is becoming increasingly apparent how much menopausal trouble arises from psychosexual causes of which many doctors are ignorant or too inhibited to discuss. And so are many of their patients, who may find women doctors more helpful here. Although these problems often arise in younger women they can persist well into and beyond middle life. They are an additional strain at the time of the climacteric which may itself precipitate or enhance them, and are at least as important as the physical manifestations of the climacteric, possibly causing even greater distress. There are a number of clinics now, some attached to hospitals, for the counselling and treatment of psychosexual problems. Women can be referred to such clinics from menopause clinics or by family doctors in the same way that gynaecological, surgical or medical referrals are made.

## Treatment

### General

Irregular vaginal bleeding with lengthening or missed periods is one indication of the approaching menopause and may be the only one in a minority of women. It should go without saying that any other cause of irregular bleeding must be excluded before a straight diagnosis of oestrogen deficiency is made. Roughly a third of all postmenopausal women who bleed from the vagina after the age of 50 have some other, perhaps more serious, condition which requires investigation. Before ovarian hormone treatment is considered, extraneous causes of bleeding have to be treated.

As well as, or before, prescribing oestrogen at the climacteric doctors often find a few simple medical measures of help. Analgesics relieve pain in muscles and joints. Hypnotics may help combat sleeplessness, while sedatives and tranquillizers are sometimes given to women who are anxious or have emotional problems. If there is bloating, or water retention, drugs which promote the flow of urine have a place in the management of the menopause.

Arguments have raged over whether tranquillizers help or hinder. They are unlikely to make life any easier for a woman with oestrogen deficiency until this has been treated but they may help thereafter and may be needed as well as oestrogen. Equally, it is unwise to take oestrogen without clear evidence of deficiency because the risks may not be justified.

## Drugs which do not contain oestrogen

Dixarit is a preparation containing clonidine, which is not a hormone, but though not as effective as oestrogen, it may be used where a woman has milder symptoms or should not be given oestrogen for a particular reason. If this drug is unsuccessful progestogens alone often help.

There has recently been some support for danazol, marketed as Danol. This lowers the level of oestrogens in the body, but also prevents the surges of hormones produced by the pituitary gland. The manufacturers have not promoted the product as suitable for menopausal conditions, but gynaecologists have noticed that when treating women with danazol for other conditions, their patients do not seem to suffer from menopausal conditions in spite of low oestrogen levels. It is being used tentatively to avoid removal of ovaries, and where oestrogen is contra-indicated because of breast conditions in some women who have menopausal symptoms.

## Prophylactic

While oestrogen is considered to be essential for women under the age of 40 whose ovaries have been removed, it is not, as already mentioned, universally recommended as a preventive for osteoporosis, although many experts believe it would be successful. It may be considered as a prophylactic in a few instances until the age of 50 in women who have had a premature menopause for no known reason, before they are 40, in view of the association of increased coronary artery disease with a premature menopause. But this decision will not be undertaken lightly without consideration of relevant factors, as in every instance where the administration of prophylactic oestrogen is under review.

## Diagnosis and assessment of oestrogen deficiency

In selecting women who may be expected to benefit from hormone treatment doctors know that if a woman is having regular periods she cannot be deficient in oestrogen. Moreover, if her periods are occurring at not more than three-monthly intervals her ovaries are probably still making enough oestrogen for her immediate needs. But if her main symptoms are hot flushes or sweats with vaginal dryness and urinary frequency the evidence is plain for all to see that she is short of oestrogen

If for a particular reason oestrogen treatment is contemplated in the absence of positive evidence of deficiency, a short trial with oestrogen therapy may sometimes be carried out. If there is no improvement in the symptoms at the end of, say, two months, it is advisable to establish that true deficiency exists before continuing treatment. Assessment of ovarian status is also important where long-term treatment is envisaged.


## The Maturation Index

Examination of the cells which line the wall of the vagina provides some indication of oestrogen deficiency and its severity. As already noted, the vagina is kept in good condition and well lubricated by the oestrogen in the body. When this supply is withdrawn, effects are seen in the lining cells of the vaginal wall. In the healthy vagina three layers of cells can be differentiated microscopically and classified according to their maturity as seen in the appearance of each layer; mature cells are on the surface, immature cells in the basal layer, and semi-immature cells in the intermediate layer.

By counting the proportion of cells of each type an index of maturity can be determined which roughly reflects the amount of oestrogen in the body. Thus a high level may give an index of 85% superficial cells, 15% intermediate cells and 0% deep cells. Lack of oestrogen may give an index of 0%, 10% and 90%.

Examination of the cells is a relatively simple procedure. The vagina is inspected through a small tube or speculum which, when introduced, holds the walls apart. Through this a little vaginal secretion is removed with a small wooden spatula which is rubbed against the side of the upper part of the vaginal wall, or the fluid may be aspirated from higher up. It is a painless exercise which may be done at the same time as a cervical smear is taken. The film can be examined directly in an out-patient department, which has the necessary staff and equipment, or it may be sent to another laboratory. New rapid staining methods have enabled slides to be prepared in a few minutes. We speak of a fully oestrogenized vaginal smear when there is a good preponderance of superficial cells, as in a healthy young woman who is menstruating regularly before the menopause. These cells are large, flat and 'cornified' with a typical nucleus. In a menopausal woman a relative absence of superficial cells may be expected, but a few intermediate and deep cells, each with a different type of nucleus, may be identified, indicating a rather feeble oestrogen effect. Although some women may retain an oestrogenized vagina well into old age – and some 40% of women over 75 show this effect – some younger women have poorly oestrogenized smears. There is wide variation from woman to woman, but after treatment with oestrogen an atrophic vaginal smear, composed predominantly of deep cells, will change and superficial cells quickly reappear. The smear gives some indication of the effect of treatment.

The vaginal cells are affected by the menstrual cycle, and in premenopausal women the smear is usually best taken around the eleventh to fourteenth day of the cycle when oestrogen values are high at ovulation. In postmenopausal women the timing is irrelevant. Other factors, including some diseases, alterations in sensitivity to body tissues, infections, drugs and hormones can affect the smear. In spite of this, and although it does not measure minor changes in the amounts of available oestrogen, this test is a good and relatively inexpensive, if crude, screening technique, but it has to be interpreted in the light of the symptoms and the clinical examination. More than a single test may be needed and serial smears often give more help.

While an atrophic vaginal smear confirms a diagnosis of oestrogen deficiency as well as providing some idea of the total oestrogen which is available, the smear has no relationship to the severity of symptoms. Some women who are experiencing flushes still show well-oestrogenized smears. It would be interesting to know if these women are the ones whose flushes respond to a placebo. More importantly it would be valuable to know if younger women with poorly oestrogenized smears are among those who are particularly at risk of developing osteoporosis later.

If accurate assessment is needed, particularly before long-term treatment is proposed, recourse can be made to more complicated blood hormone levels including oestrogen. High pituitary hormone levels correspond with the appearance of vaginal dryness and hot flushes, and the levels fall sharply when the symptoms are alleviated by hormone treatment. But here again the results must be interpreted in conjunction with a woman's symptoms and her doctor's clinical examination, and serial analyses may be necessary. Unfortunately the values overlap in premenopausal women, and so do not provide absolute criteria. These very expensive endocrinological tests are not at present practicable for all women who receive hormone treatment. Though they have proved valuable in much-needed research, they are rarely required in practice.

## Treatment regimes

Oestrogen may be given for the immediate relief of symptoms arising at the time of the normal menopause, for a premature menopause whether natural or artificial on a long-term basis, or as a prophylactic. The regimes differ according to need, symptoms and the individual requirement as determined by the prescribing doctor.

*Short-term treatment* aims to provide oestrogen for as long as symptoms persist without it, in the smallest effective dose which will control them. But too short a period is demoralizing when symptoms return. Most gynaecologists expect that at least one to two years' treatment will be needed. Each doctor employs his own criteria, dose, type of hormone, alone or in combination, as well as the route by which treatment is to be given. Women are not all alike and differ in response to and need for treatment. Once it has been decided to stop treatment oestrogen is withdrawn slowly over a period of months to avoid a flare-up of symptoms. Doctors usually halve and then quarter the dose until, in the absence of symptoms, the treatment is finally stopped altogether.

*Long-term treatment* may be advised if symptoms persist unduly. It is considered essential for women who have had their ovaries removed under the age of 40. This requires regular supervision. As already discussed, arguments have been advanced in favour of giving oestrogens in order to prevent osteoporosis developing after the menopause, and a woman in whose family – her mother perhaps – osteoporosis has been troublesome may be considered as a suitable candidate if she appears to be oestrogen-deficient and there are no contra-indications. The dose of oestrogen required to control osteoporosis is higher than that needed for atrophic vaginitis which may respond to 0.3 mg conjugated oestrogens, while for osteoporosis it may be necessary to give more than 1.25 mg. Prophylactic oestrogen may sometimes be considered until they are 50 for women whose periods have ceased before they are 40 in view of the association of increased coronary disease with a premature menopause.

### Choice of oestrogen

Natural oestrogens occur in the living tissues of man and animals; synthetic oestrogens are made in the laboratory. Natural oestrogens occur as oestrone, oestradiol and oestriol, and as conjugates such as equine oestrogen, oestrone sulphate, oestriol glucuronide. But recent research at King's College Hospital and the Chelsea Hospital for Women indicates that when taken by mouth these are virtually all converted to oestrone. Natural oestrogens may be made by biological extraction and purification, or in the laboratory by attachment to a carrier which splits off in the intestine leaving the natural oestrogen to be absorbed as oestrone. Examples are piperazine oestrone sulphate, oestradiol valerate, and oestriol succinate. Synthetic oestrogens are made from either natural or entirely synthetic precursors. The main synthetics are ethinyloestradiol, mestranol, diesnoestrol, and stilboestrol. These do not occur in living tissues but have similar actions to the oestrogens which are made in the body. But whereas natural oestrogens raise the oestrogens in the blood, the synthetic oestrogens circulate unchanged, and are not metabolized to the three main oestrogens.

**Properties of oestrogens**

Conjugated oestrogens are soluble in water, and when taken by mouth are more active than free oestrogens, are not so readily destroyed by the liver, and are therefore more potent. Natural free oestrogens are soluble in oil, relatively weak when given by mouth, but active by injection. Semi-synthetic oestrogens made from natural oestrogens are active when given by mouth and have some side effects, although less in lower doses. The other synthetics are active by mouth, and may have substantial side effects. The latter preparations are considerably cheaper to produce. There is some evidence suggesting that the so-called natural oestrogens do not cause a rise in triglycerides unlike some synthetic compounds, nor do they affect the blood pressure. It is likely that the use of natural oestrogens may reduce the chances of thrombosis and other side effects occurring as a result of treatment, but much of the speculation on this subject has been generated by the scarcity of scientific evidence and the enthusiasm of the pharmaceutical houses in promoting their own products. The effects of all oestrogens are probably related to the dose, especially in the case of synthetic oestrogens. These are now given in much lower doses than formerly.

**Administration**

Oestrogen may be given in the following ways:

1 By mouth
2 By injection into a muscle or vein

3 As a depot or implant, from which the hormones are slowly released over a period of months

4 By local application into the vagina

## 1 Oestrogen by mouth

When taken by mouth oestrogen may be given continuously or cyclically. In the latter method the hormone is taken for twenty-one days, followed by seven days when the tablets are not taken. Gynaecologists now tend to prefer continuous treatment because symptoms may recur in the treatment-free week, which was advocated to 'rest' the endometrium and avoid overstimulation. This is now usually effected by the addition of a progestogen in the seven treatment-free days – sequential treatment – or by giving a progestogen for a week to ten days in each calendar month of continuous oestrogen-combined treatment.

In premenopausal women bleeding occurs at the end of the 'rest' period and is known as withdrawal bleeding, and some postmenopausal women may also bleed in this way. Bleeding which occurs during the twenty-one treatment days is known as 'break-through' bleeding. It is troublesome in about 40% of menopausal women, and is usually due either to underdosage or overdosage of oestrogen. If it is not controlled on reducing or increasing the dose aspiration of the endometrial contents is usually required in order to find out why. This is done by examining the fluid and cells of the endometrial lining microscopically. This method is used to screen women for changes brought about by overstimulation of the endometrium either by administered oestrogens, or when the amount made in the body is high. Samples of uterine cells were formerly obtained by dilatation and curettage which requires a general anaesthetic. A more simple method can be carried out in an out-patient department without an anaesthetic, thanks to the development of a method of aspiration using a small steel curette, the Vabra curette, which is about 3mm in diameter. These curettes can usually be easily passed through the cervix. About 4% of women find this uncomfortable. As a patient myself, I have found the newer Isaacs aspirator can be inserted without discomfort. These techniques constitute a major break-through in the care of menopausal women. All women on treatment, especially without a progestogen, are advised to have these examinations regularly to monitor any changes in the endometrium.

*Rationale of addition of a progestogen.* It will be remembered that in the natural menstrual cycle a surge of progesterone takes place following ovulation. This alters the endometrium from the stage in which the glands proliferate and the endometrium thickens to the stage described as secretory. At the end of this stage the progesterone-induced menstrual flow begins, and the endometrium returns to its premenstrual condition. Progesterone in nature counteracts the changes brought about by the proliferative action of oestrogen. When taken by mouth as treatment the synthetic progestogen has the similar clinical effect of reversing the stimulatory effect of oestrogen. By bringing on a scheduled bleed as in a normal period it ensures that the lining of the endometrium is shed. This progestogen-induced regular bleeding is the price which has to be paid for a better control of symptoms of menopausal distress and for greater safety in treatment. Some postmenopausal women may have difficulty in at first accepting a return to monthly bleeding after the age at which the periods have ceased.

About 5% of women on treatment voluntarily stop taking oestrogen; another 5% decline to start, but nine out of ten post-menopausal women are willing to put up with bleeding for the sake of the concomitant advantages, even though some have been known to practise some dissimulation when purchasing their tampons ostensibly for their daughters, rather than acquire the label of a 'menstruating granny'. The bleeding is often only a smear – its onset is predictable, almost to the hour – and it can be manipulated to fit in with social or other plans by varying the date on which the progestogen is taken. These 'periods' do not indicate a return of fertility.

Progesterone can sometimes have a somewhat depressant action, and some women do not feel as well while they are

114

taking it, usually depending on the dose. Some progestogens cause swelling or shrinkage of breast tissue, sometimes induce a little spotting, and occasionally virilization, but progesterone has considerable importance in treatment. On its own it has some effect on flushing, but the great advantage lies in its ability to balance some of the effects of overstimulation by producing an anti-oestrogen enzyme, and preventing unduly high oestrogen levels reaching individual nuclei in cells. For premenopausal women whose periods are irregular or prolonged, progesterone often settles the bleeding into a more regular pattern.

The pharmaceutical industry has shown considerable ingenuity in marketing pack preparations for hormone treatment in a form women find convenient to use according to the effect required by the doctor. The newer packs simplify the problem for the woman who may be forgetful or even confused. A missed pill should be remedied by taking two pills the following day.

*Premarin*, which is one of the longest-established preparations, consists of conjugated oestrogen – that is natural oestrogen – derived from the urine of pregnant mares. It contains a high proportion of sodium equilin sulphate, a potent equine hormone, and other unspecified oestrogens including oestrone sulphate, the form in which oestradiol, the principal follicular hormone, is excreted. It comes in four different strengths coloured accordingly. Green, red, yellow or purple tablets contain 0.3 mg, 0.625 mg, 1.25 mg and 2.5 mg respectively. It is recommended by the manufacturers as suitable for short- or long-term treatment. The progestogen can be added on the seven tablet-free days.

*Harmogen* is piperazine oestrone sulphate, a so-called natural oestrogen made in one-strength tablets of 1.5 mg. The manufacturers recommend that one tablet should be taken twice a day adjusted to the lowest dose needed to control symptoms for which one tablet a day could be adequate. It can be taken cyclically or continuously, according to the wishes of the prescriber.

115

*Progynova* is oestradiol valerate, also a natural oestrogen. It was the first twenty-one-day pack marketed for the menopause. There are two tablet strengths, 2 mg and 1 mg, the 2 mg being recommended for initial therapy followed by seven tablet-free days until a satisfactory response is obtained. The dose can then be reduced and continued for up to six weeks (two packs) after which seven tablet-free days follow. It is suitable for short courses of treatment.

*Mixogen*, *Climatone* and *Mepilin* are oral preparations in which the synthetic ethinyloestradiol is combined with a male sex hormone, methyltestosterone, of which a small amount is converted to oestradiol. These preparations may be helpful for women in whom sexual desire is decreased, but may cause some downy facial hair after prolonged treatment, and they may also not control flushing as well as other preparations.

*Ethinyloestradiol* is also available in straight tablet form in doses of 10 to 20 microgrammes given daily. A progestogen can be added separately in treatment, which is usually given cyclically.

To avoid giving a separate dose of progestogen in the last half of the treatment cycle, so-called 'sequential' regimes have been introduced.

*Syntex Menophase* combines mestranol, and the progestogen norethisterone. This product is among those more recently introduced for the treatment of the menopause, and comes in a bubble pack of twenty-eight tablets. It comprises six different formulations, each coloured by its label. Thus five pink, eight orange, two yellow, three green, six blue and four lavender tablets have been elaborated to follow as closely as possible the equivalent hormonal stages of the twenty-eight-day menstrual cycle. This is intended to eliminate the possibility of resurgence of symptoms sometimes encountered in the week-off treatment in cyclical unopposed therapy. The green, blue and lavender tablets each contain the progestogen norethisterone. The woman takes her first tablet on any suitable day – the manufacturers suggest Sunday – and takes one at the same time each day, following the arrows round the pack for twenty-eight days.

*Cycloprogynova* similarly combines the two hormones in a sequential form and consists of a combination of the natural oestrogen oestradiol valerate and the progestogen norgestrel and is recommended by the manufacturers for long-term use. The hormones are formulated in a cyclical manner by eleven white tablets each containing 2 mg of oestradiol valerate, and ten orange tablets of 0.5 mg of the progestogen norgestrel. This provides seven tablet-free days. The manufacturers advise that Cycloprogynova is not an oral contraceptive in spite of its ingredients, and say that oral contraceptives should not be taken at the same time.

*Prempak*, recently introduced, comprises twenty-one tablets of Premarin, either 0.625 mg or 1.25 mg, with seven tablets of 0.5 mg of dinorgestrel.

## 2 Oestrogen by injection

The advantages of this are limited to the use of preparations which are inactivated in the stomach and to women who suffer from malabsorption conditions. The treatment has ceased to find much support today.

## 3 Hormone implants

Depot hormone release is an old method of replacement which fell from favour, but enthusiasm has revived. The use of oestrogen implants gives good results and seems likely to be extended. An implant has an added advantage over having to take a pill every day, in that the oestrogen released over months from a depot does not pass through the liver, which eliminates the possibility of toxic action by breakdown products. Having a pellet inserted is a painless and simple procedure which takes only a few minutes, and many women prefer to have their oestrogen

117

given in this way, especially if they are forgetful or nauseated by oestrogen by mouth.

*Technique for insertion of implants.* The pellet is usually placed in the layer of fat just under the skin of the abdominal wall, or the skin of the buttock. A local anaesthetic is first introduced into a sterilized area of skin, and a small tube or trochar with a sharp point and an inner rod is passed through the skin to the required depth. The rod is withdrawn and a pellet of either 2 mm or 4.5 mm diameter is dropped down the outer tube. The tube is then withdrawn and the skin covered with a dressing which has to be kept dry for forty-eight hours. A 25 or 50 mg pellet of oestradiol lasts about six months and a 100 mg one approximately nine months before symptoms recur, and women know as soon as they begin to need another implant.

The pellet usually begins to work after a week, quickly relieves flushing, and usually vaginal atrophic symptoms too, but the implant technique is particularly suited to women who suffer from loss of libido or sexual drive which does not respond to oestrogen unless it is due to or associated with vaginal dryness causing painful intercourse. A supplementary implant of 100 mg of testosterone, a male sex hormone, almost always improves libido within six weeks, although this symptom is usually the first to recur as the effect on climacteric symptoms returns as the pellet becomes used up. The method is useful for women who have severe psychosexual or marital problems.

The accompanying table illustrates the effect of treatment by implant on sexual function. It is based on the results in 35 women followed for three to nine months after treatment with a mixed implant of oestradiol and testosterone, 20 who were given oestradiol alone and 7 who received testosterone alone. Testosterone alone was given only to 7 women, since although it significantly affects sexual drive it does not improve climacteric symptoms. As the table shows, oestradiol has only a marginal effect on libido (although it is very effective in controlling other climacteric symptoms), but a significant improvement in sexual function occurred in the majority of the 37 women who had mixed implants.

| Libido response to different regimes of hormone implants | | | | | |
|---|---|---|---|---|---|
| Implants | Duration of therapy (months) | Sexual interest Absent | Weak | Moderate | Strong |
| **Oestradiol** 50mg/ | 0 (pretherapy) | 14 | 4 | 0 | 0 |
| 100mg=20 | 3 - 9 | 12 | 6 | 2 | 0 |
| **Testosterone** 200mg=7 | 0 (pretherapy) | 5 | 2 | 0 | 0 |
| | 6 - 9 | 1 | 1 | 3 | 2 |
| **Oestradiol** + 50mg | 0 (pretherapy) | 30 | 5 | 0 | 0 |
| **Testosterone** 100mg=35 | 3 - 9 | 0 | 7 | 20 | 7 |

From *The Menopause* (Clinics in Obstetrics and Gynaecology. Vol 4, No 1), guest editors Robert B. Greenblatt and John Studd.

The implant technique was originally introduced many years ago for women whose ovaries had been removed and its use is likely to be restored to favour for young women without ovaries. The reason why gynaecologists have previously avoided this simple and effective method of hormone treatment is that it tends to produce irregular bleeding. This can, however, be regulated by progesterone, and women who have had an implant are now advised to take 5 mg of norethisterone by mouth for the first seven or more days of each calendar month. A scheduled regular scanty bleed follows on the eighth day. If a woman fails to take a progestogen, overstimulation of the lining of the uterus and heavy vaginal bleeding will follow. Gynaecologists will usually not put in an implant for anyone who has not had a hysterectomy unless she can be relied on to take progestogen for at least seven days each month if so instructed.

Testosterone should not be taken by women who are unduly hairy because it tends to increase the growth of hair on the face, and this was noticed by four women in the series to which the table refers. Testosterone may sometimes deepen the voice and encourage the development of acne in postmenopausal women.

## 4 Oestrogen applied locally

Vaginal atrophy responds well to oestrogen given in one of the usual ways by mouth. If, however, a woman has no symptoms other than vaginal dryness, or if oestrogen by mouth does not entirely relieve painful intercourse, a jelly such as KY or dienoestrol cream may be used with an applicator inserted directly into the vagina daily for a month, and then used two or three times a week for two months, or longer if necessary. Oestrogen pessaries are also available.

Premarin vaginal cream contains 0.625 mg per gram of conjugated oestrogens in a non-liquefying base. A calibrated applicator is supplied with the pack.

Application of oestrogen cream often helps to relieve the annoying itchiness of the perineal skin at the climacteric and is sometimes prescribed with hydrocortisone ointment. Owing to the sensitivity of the vagina to oestrogen the latter is absorbed rapidly, and larger doses have produced vaginal bleeding. Occasionally overgrowth of the endometrium has been recorded following vaginal administration in large doses, and a progestogen by mouth may be prescribed in addition for women who use oestrogen locally in this way.

## Side effects of hormone therapy

I have already referred to rare side effects of progestogens. About 10% of women develop side effects during oestrogen treatment. A very sensitive sign of overdosage with oestrogen is breast discomfort. Nausea, vomiting, lack of appetite, bloating and sometimes vaginal discharge do occur, but they may also occur on a placebo as well as on active preparations of oestrogen. When mild, these symptoms usually disappear on their own, usually within a few weeks. If they persist, the dose of oestrogen is reduced until one which is acceptable to the woman is discovered, or the preparation may be changed by trial and error to one which suits the woman better. There may also be an increase in weight, and some women develop freckles.

Nausea may be helped by taking the pills after meals. If bloating continues it may be relieved by a diuretic such as Lasix which promotes the flow of urine. Lasix is often given with additional potassium which is present in fresh orange or pineapple juice, or as tablets.

*Frequency of side effects.* Some idea of the frequency of side effects can be obtained from the figures given by John Studd and his colleagues in 112 women treated for six months. Of these, breast tenderness occurred in 20 women. It was considered a minor complaint, being more noticeable in the latter part of the cycle, and was possibly due to the progesterone. 10 women complained of nausea, mainly restricted to the first treatment cycle. 2 women had superficial thrombosis in the legs. 15 discontinued the treatment, about the same as the proportion of women who stop taking the Pill.

After six months' treatment with oestrogen for three weeks out of four, there was very considerable improvement as can be seen in the table below. Depression fell in from 66.6% to 27%

Presenting symptoms in 60 premenopausal patients attending the menopause clinic with apparent climacteric symptoms. The symptomatic response to 1.25 mg of Premarin over six months is shown.

| Symptoms | Pre-treatment (n=60) | | After 6 months' oestrogen therapy (n=56) | |
|---|---|---|---|---|
| | No | % | No | % |
| Hot flushes | 25 | 41.6 | 7 | 12.5 |
| Insomnia | 27 | 45.0 | 7 | 12.5 |
| Depression | 40 | 66.6 | 15 | 27.0 |
| Headaches | 31 | 50.0 | 11 | 19.8 |
| Dyspareunia | 12 | 20.0 | 1 | 1.8 |
| Loss of libido | 25 | 41.6 | 21 | 37.8 |
| Aches and pains | 27 | 45.0 | 13 | 23.4 |
| Poor concentration | 36 | 60.0 | 13 | 23.4 |
| Irritability | 44 | 73.3 | 21 | 37.8 |

From *The Menopause* (Clinics in Obstetrics and Gynaecology. Vol 4, No 1), guest editors Robert B. Greenblatt and John Studd.

of women, poor concentration in from 60% to 23.4%, headaches in from 50% to 19.8%, and insomnia in from 45% to 12.5%. But the greatest improvement occurred in the women who had had dyspareunia or painful intercourse, which fell from 20% to 1.8% on treatment.

The least improvement occurred in women who had found their sex drive or libido diminished, as might be expected because oestrogen alone exerts comparatively little effect here – unlike its effect on atrophic vaginitis, where it constitutes replacement of a deficient supply of oestrogen.

## Results of treatment
## Flushes

Flushes at the menopause, or the vasomotor symptoms of impaired tension in blood vessels, correspond to pituitary hormone levels, and the same phenomenon has been found in men whose testes have been surgically removed. These men too may then experience hot flushes accompanied by high pituitary hormone levels, which fall as do women's when the appropriate hormone is administered. Since we can measure the number of hot flushes we can also measure the effect of treatment. Flushes almost always disappear or are greatly improved when oestrogen is given, and their frequency and duration diminish, though it should be remembered that they may also respond to a placebo. The symptoms are usually improved within fifteen days of receiving oestrogen and this is followed later by a return to nearly normal pituitary hormone levels.

Many investigators have tried to find out how long flushing may last if untreated. One survey in England has shown that of the 75% of menopausal women who had experienced hot flushes, these lasted over a year in four out of five sufferers, and for more than five years in over a quarter. In some untreated women flushing may last for many years while other women find the flushes pass in a few months. Probably the peak in the frequency of flushing occurs about two years after the last menstrual period.

Almost half a group of menopausal women when questioned found flushing caused them acute discomfort, and one in five said the flush alone was embarrassing. There is therefore a good reason for treating all women who suffer severe inconvenience and distress until such time as the flushing fails to begin again when they stop treatment. A minority of women, perhaps 5% to 10%, may require treatment on a longer-term basis.

## Genital symptoms

These symptoms too are probably much commoner than we have realized, either because a woman may be too shy to talk about them or may not realize they too are due to oestrogen deficiency. They almost always immediately respond to treatment with oestrogen in lower doses than are required for vasomotor symptoms.

## Loss of libido

In the controversy as to the advisability or otherwise of giving oestrogens to menopausal women, gynaecologists do not dispute the important role of oestrogen in the management of both hot flushes and dyspareunia. The question as to whether loss of libido or sex drive is a direct effect of oestrogen deprivation is not so easily agreed. There seems no doubt that many women do experience a lack of interest in sexual relations at the climacteric, but this may be a side effect of dyspareunia, or part of a psychological process affected by extraneous influences which oestrogen will not relieve and which may call for psychotherapy.

The table on page 124 gives the details of the symptoms other than flushing, experienced by a group of women, together with their response to oestrogen. Here dramatic improvement in painful intercourse resulted, producing further evidence of the sensitivity of the vagina to oestrogen. The same table shows that all symptoms returned when oestrogen was stopped after six months. Before treatment 55% of women were depressed and only 11% after treatment, but depression returned in 46% on stopping oestrogen; 38% of women had insomnia before, 2% after treatment, but 41% on stopping treatment. Dyspareunia improved from 24% before to 2% after treatment, with a return to 13% on stopping treatment. Joint pains improved from 20% to 7% and increased to 26% of women when treatment was stopped. Poor libido improved temporarily from 20% to 4% and returned to 13%.

Percentage of patients presenting with symptoms before, during and after treatment with Syntex Menophase.

| Symptom | Pre-treat-ment | 2 months' treat-ment | 4 months' treat-ment | 6 months' treat-ment | Post-treat-ment |
|---|---|---|---|---|---|
| Depression/anxiety | 55 | 18 | 14 | 11 | 46 |
| Insomnia | 38 | 5 | 3 | 2 | 41 |
| Lethargy | 30 | 8 | 4 | – | 31 |
| Dyspareunia | 24 | 11 | 1 | 2 | 13 |
| Headache | 22 | 10 | 8 | 9 | 26 |
| Reduced libido | 20 | 14 | 6 | 4 | 13 |
| Joint pains & backache | 20 | 12 | 12 | 7 | 26 |
| Poor concentration | 19 | 5 | – | – | 13 |

From *The Menopause* (Clinics in Obstetrics and Gynaecology. Vol 4, No 1), guest editors Robert B. Greenblatt and John Studd.

## Summary

As we have seen, oestrogen almost invariably relieves sweating and flushing in a week or two. The vagina is lubricated in about two weeks, with improvement in urinary symptoms. It may take six weeks for sex drive or libido to return, and this does not always improve. But numbers of women have paid tribute to the transformation hormone treatment has made in their lives. They say they feel completely different and experience a new feeling of well-being, with a return in interest and efficiency. Once this has restored their confidence they are able to cope where before they were just muddling through. 'Fantastic' is not too strong a description to apply to some of the results of treatment.

These are some of the remarks I have heard in menopause clinics:

'I don't get any flushes now. I don't feel hot in bed. And I'm less depressed. Sex is OK now.'

'Since my implant I feel I can cope with things. The vagina is less dry and I am getting orgasms as I did before all the trouble started, before I came here. I do notice I'm a bit more hairy than before.'

'My husband's a very happy man, now.'

'When I stopped taking the tablets I got forgetful again after about four weeks. I read about this treatment in a magazine and now I feel absolutely marvellous.'

'If I get short with my daughter or my husband they say, "Haven't you taken your pill yet?" '

'We were down to having intercourse once a year. I used to think "O crikey" and put him off. Now it's about once a month.'

'My husband tells his friends to send their wives here.'

'I had heavy periods with discharge. I used to go all hot twice a day. I had terrible headaches and used to cry all the time. And then there was terrible vaginal irritation. All that has gone.'

'It was lack of sleep that made me come here. Since I've been having treatment we both sleep now.'

'The flushes went in two weeks, but sometimes they come back during the week I'm not taking the tablets. I used to wake up wringing wet and fling open the windows. My husband thought he'd get pneumonia if I didn't get something done about it. He'd read about the menopause in *She.*'

'I'd had one ovary removed, and I was getting flushes every half-hour. I'd feel very restless before they came on. And irritable, you've no idea, shouting at the kids and the poor man if they crossed my path. The flushes went in two weeks on treatment.'

'I'd been on Valium, but I was still tense and I couldn't sleep.'

'I was always in tears, nobody dared speak to me and my concentration was very bad. It's coming back now.'

'I had Premarin for my flushes. They were coming every

fifteen minutes with aches and pains and insomnia and headaches. The lot. They've all improved and apart from the bleeding I'm OK.'

'I went to the doctor *so many times* and just said how low I felt. I had no sex drive and it was painful with my husband. I'd been like it for three years. The doctor just told me to go and see some sex films in the West End. At the clinic first I had Premarin and the flushes went. Now that I've had an implant I'm back to a young woman again. We have intercourse once or twice a week now. We'd had none for three years while I was on ice. I did get some breast tenderness but it's gone now, though I think the implant is wearing off.'

'A blind comes down, and you feel like cold meat. We did everything to relax me; even tried drink. It's been fantastic since I came here. My husband nearly had a nervous breakdown over my sexual coldness.'

'I'd had panic feelings and sweats and headaches. I'd had them for eight years. Since I've had Progynova I only get about one flush a day and perhaps another at night. I get a white discharge, but I've stopped taking the tablets now. The symptoms aren't bad enough.'

'My memory is better. My family think I'm more intelligent now. And my joints haven't ached so much since I started on Harmogen.'

'I'd like to carry on with the tablets. I feel more like *me*, the one I used to be.'

'My periods stopped when I was 50. I had no interest in sex and I found my husband hard to talk to. My depression improved with the tablets.'

'I could never make anyone take any interest in me. I might have got worse if I hadn't made the doctor send me here. I expect he's told you I read about it in the *News of the World*.'

'I don't like tablets. I'd rather have the symptoms.'

'I've not been a joy to be with since I ran out of Premarin.'

'I don't even think about my age now.'

'After the first month of treatment I began to feel I was ticking over again. But I don't feel so good on the week off.'

126

'I do have a weight problem on treatment. But it's worth it to be more efficient now, although being an actress it's also a disadvantage if you put on a few pounds.'

# 9 The risks of hormone treatment

For all its many advantages, oestrogen, like all powerful drugs, carries the potential to harm. It would be surprising if it did not, especially if used in the wrong way. Risks are, in any case, always relative, and all medicine is a balancing of one risk against another. Common sense demands that benefit must outweigh the risk in medical care. For a woman whose life is made utterly miserable by her menopausal condition slightly greater risks may justifiably be taken in her treatment. We are all more cautious about the indiscriminate use of oestrogen now, including American doctors who have had longer experience in treating women with it, and have had to learn some hard lessons. The long-term trials which are now in progress on both sides of the Atlantic are already bearing fruit in throwing further light on the safety of the treatment, as well as on the adverse effects which have been reported recently.

There are some situations which carry risks which do not justify the treatment, particularly those conditions which oestrogen exacerbates. On the other hand, there are lesser risks which require cautious appraisal, but which do not necessarily contra-indicate the use of oestrogen. Her gynaecologist or general practitioner may consider that one or more of the following conditions make it inadvisable for a woman to take oestrogen, but will in addition have to weigh up other factors such as her past medical history, the severity of her symptoms and the degree of necessary supervision. An outsider is in no position to give an opinion here. Each woman's case must be judged individually.

**Lower risk factors**

*1 High blood pressure.* Oestrogens, particularly the synthetic oestrogens, can raise the blood pressure, and a woman who already has a blood pressure which is higher than normal may have to avoid taking oestrogen. If she is already taking drugs which lower blood pressure she will probably require closer scrutiny and will be kept under regular observation if oestrogen is prescribed in addition. This also goes for a woman in whom the blood pressure was known to have been unduly high during a pregnancy.

2 *Obesity*. When assessing the advisability of giving oestrogen to a woman who is overweight doctors will recall that a precursor is converted into oestrogen in the fatty tissues of the body and fat women are liable to produce higher amounts of oestrogen themselves. This is carried in the bloodstream into the nucleus of the cells of the endometrium and may result in its overstimulation. A woman who cannot reduce excessive weight may be the wrong candidate for oestrogen.

3 *Lipids*. Because of the association of fat and arterial conditions, women who have unduly high blood fats are usually considered to be unsuitable for oestrogen treatment. This is based on the rise in one type (triglycerides) which oestrogens, particularly synthetic oestrogens, can cause in the blood. In this context the association of smoking with heart conditions may preclude the administration of oestrogens to women who smoke heavily, particularly if they are already at risk on account of concomitant factors.

4 *Gall stones*. It is known that women who take oestrogen run a two-and-a-half-fold increased chance of developing gall stones. For this reason a woman who has had a recent attack of gall bladder disease, such as cholecystitis, or a woman who already has gall stones may be advised not to have prolonged oestrogen treatment.

5 *Diabetes*. People who suffer from diabetes are less able to deal with sugar than non-diabetics. As a result the levels of sugar in their blood may be too high unless they take insulin. Oestrogen reduces the body's capacity to deal with glucose, probably by affecting the activity of the insulin produced by the body. The

levels of blood sugar in women on the contraceptive pill are often above normal, and the same effect has been noted in some young women whose ovaries have been removed and who are being treated with oestrogen. Theoretically, taking oestrogen could accelerate the rate at which diabetes and its associated incidence of atherosclerosis could arise in menopausal women. In fact, 19% of the women who attended the Birmingham menopause clinic already had some mild alteration in the ability to metabolize sugar before treatment. After the group had been treated for six months with a synthetic oestrogen the figure had risen to 38%, but none became frankly diabetic. John Studd confirmed this, but found no change using natural hormones.

Fortunately glucose tolerance returns to normal in most younger women on discontinuing the Pill. Further research may clarify the position with regard to the postmenopausal woman on hormone treatment. Until then, and because one type of diabetes may arise in older women at the age when the natural stores of oestrogen are vanishing, there seems no logical reason to withhold oestrogen from diabetic women, unless a physician advises otherwise, provided their diabetes is carefully controlled by regular blood sugar and urine examinations, a normal precaution in any diabetic person.

## Higher risk factors

*1 Liver disease.* Hormones are carried round the body in the blood before being excreted in the urine. During this process they pass directly through the liver after being absorbed in the intestine when taken by mouth and are broken down, the liver acting as a chemical factory. If the liver is in any way damaged, the metabolism is likely to be impaired and some breakdown products then have toxic effects. Very occasionally, in addition to exerting such toxicity on the body they have induced malignant changes in the liver. Consequently women who have severe liver disease, or those who have had a recent attack of jaundice are usually considered unsuitable for hormone treatment until the tests of liver function, which may have to be repeated, return to normal.

*2 Thrombosis.* The chances of thrombosis, or clotting of blood, in the veins of arteries increases with advancing age as the circulation slows down, and a woman who has had a recent severe vein thrombosis with swelling and pain, usually in the leg, or has had a cerebral or coronary thrombosis should not run the risk of exaggerating her tendency to bloodclots by taking oestrogen. Many surgeons advise their patients to stop taking oestrogens for a month before 'cold' surgery or planned operations, in order to minimize the risk of deep vein thrombosis or pulmonary embolism after the operation.

*3 Tumours.* Some tumours grow faster in the presence of oestrogen, and are then said to be 'oestrogen-dependent'. Certain breast tumours fall into this category and if they are in existence at the time oestrogen is given are more readily disseminated. One type of tumour of the uterus is also oestrogen-dependent, and so is one sort of ovarian condition. It would be illogical, let alone dangerous, for a woman who has an oestrogen-dependent tumour to take oestrogen. The problem which only clinicians can solve for each woman who has had such a tumour removed is whether or not to allow her to take oestrogen afterwards. A past history of pelvic disease such as fibroids or endometriosis poses a similar problem for the doctor, in that both these conditions may be reactivated by oestrogen.

# 10 The cancer issue

At the centre of the problems associated with treatment of menopausal distress is the nagging medical fear and public suspicion that oestrogens may cause cancer. There is now little doubt that an association as far as the uterus is concerned exists *when the hormone is given inappropriately.* We do not know the extent of that risk, but some gynaecologists believe it has been exaggerated and statisticians tend to remain sceptical. The resulting uncertainty is disturbing, and unless it is soon resolved it may limit the use of hormones for women who are in need of treatment. As it is, British women are under- rather than over-treated. Of the three to four million women who are aged 48 to 58 probably only about a fifth of those who need treatment receive it.

We are witnessing the swing of the pendulum from one era which, at least in America, promised women the postponement of the physical loss of femininity, to an era which may be in danger of denying the needy treatment. At the same time, because it has such a spectacular effect when used correctly for the right woman, there is still a danger that oestrogen may become the sort of over-used and much abused panacea that tranquillizers were in the sixties.

The cancer scare has been the subject of extensive reporting in the national press on both sides of the Atlantic, some of it uninformed. It has also provided material for numerous papers and editorials in medical journals, some arriving at different conclusions, and in the case of editorials, offering contrary advice and opinions in the same journal on separate dates. It is fair though to say that medical opinion is moving from speculation as to risk, to consideration of the best way to minimize and ultimately eliminate any risk. The argument is not over, and this has confused many family doctors on whom devolves the obligation to protect their patients.

The scare arose in 1975 when the influential *New England Journal of Medicine* published the findings of a group of American doctors who reported an unexpectedly high rate of cancer of the endometrium, or cancer of the body of the uterus, in women who had received oestrogen treatment at the climacteric. The ensuing controversy, and the other reports which soon followed, failed to establish the extent of the link, but some of the far-reaching research which has since been instigated in Britain appears to confirm some suspicions raised in America.

The difficulty has been that the initial approach to the problem was misleading. This depended on identifying from their hospital records a number of American women who had been diagnosed as suffering from endometrial cancer. The next step was to see which of these women had taken oestrogens and which had not, and compare the two groups. A large proportion of women with cancer were alleged to have taken oestrogen, some for many years, but in many instances the dosage and duration of treatment, and even in some cases the diagnosis, was in doubt. Statistical criteria had not always been properly applied in comparing the two groups. The difficulty was increased by the fallibility of human memory in assessing incomplete records in retrospect, and by the tendency in the past to take oestrogen in doses which we now know were unsafe, and were almost certainly taken by women without regular supervision. Cancer may already have been established before the treatment was erroneously given to some women, but was mistakenly later attributed to treatment. It is not surprising that early records gave rise to considerable doubts as to their validity.

In Britain we have been able to learn many lessons from America. We have not adopted the retrospective approach. Our research looks forward and aims to follow the course of events in women from the time they first take oestrogen in known doses and regimes, not *after* they may have developed early side effects or even malignant changes. In this way changes can be picked up in time at an early stage, and all treatment monitored.

This is not to say that all retrospective studies are of no value. The highly respected epidemiologists, Professors Sir Richard Doll and Martin Vessey, and their colleagues at Oxford have observed that the risks of the order recorded in some American studies seldom prove to be artefacts. In one study in Los Angeles the risk of endometrial cancer was claimed to be increased four, seven, and nearly fourteen times, the longer oestrogen was taken before the cancer was diagnosed. In another, probably better-documented, study in Southern California, the risk of taking oestrogen was reported as having increased eight times with all oestrogens, and five times with conjugated oestrogens. *But*, virtually no women in the small community studied had taken a progestogen, and many had taken oestrogens continuously without a treatment-free week each month.

Although according to our own statistics there has been no increase in the UK as yet – and it is still early – several cancer registries in the USA recorded notable increases in endometrial cancer over the period 1963 to 1974. In an effort to find a path through what one American editorial writer aptly described as the 'Estrogen-Cancer Maze' the American Food and Drugs Administration held its own investigation into the 1975/76 reports, during which one editorial in *Drug Therapy* noted in February 1976: 'The statistical analyses of clinical data have gotten so cryptic that the people who know what the results mean cannot articulate them, and the people who could articulate them don't know what they mean.' Not a bad summary. The investigating committee finally decided that no real conclusions could be reached at that stage, but the FDA later made an order which requires drug manufacturers to include in oestrogen packaging, guidelines and warnings for doctors regarding endometrial cancer.

It must now be accepted that there is no smoke without fire, and this is borne out by some evidence which is already available.

## Animal experiments

Tumours have been produced experimentally in specially bred mice by giving them oestrogen, though without a progestogen. Similarly, endometrial cancer has been induced by injecting rabbits with synthetic oestrogen. Few experts would deny that large doses of oestrogen unopposed by a progestogen can eventually cause overgrowth of the endometrium which, if prolonged, may progress to pre- or frank malignancy. The overgrowth can usually be reversed by stopping the oestrogen or by adding a progestogen. Oestrogens are 'primers' or growth stimulants in this respect.

## Clinical experience

Postmenopausal women who have tumours which themselves produce oestrogen are reported to have more chances of getting endometrial cancer. Fat women are three to nine times more liable to do so than thin women. Here, the reason is likely to be that an oestrogen precursor is changed in fat to oestrogen. After the menopause this provides the main source of oestrogen as oestrone (the follicles have stopped producing oestradiol). Women who develop endometrial cancer convert more precursors and so have higher levels of oestrone in their blood. This can be further raised by medication because it is now believed that oestradiol when taken by mouth changes to oestrone after it has been absorbed from the intestine. The significance of these high blood levels is that oestrone is probably the strongest stimulator of overgrowth or hyperplasia of the endometrium.

Moreover, these large amounts of oestrone gain access to the nucleus of the endometrial cells by a special mechanism which further elevates the amount of oestrone reaching each cell via the bloodstream. It is at this point that progesterone acts to counteract the effect of oestrogen within the cell nucleus. In nearly all the American studies reporting an increase in endometrial cancer, no progestogen had been given. This is clearly an important aspect in considering the relationship between oestrogen and cancer.

## Diagnosis

Endometrial cancer causes no symptoms in its early stages in 20% of cases, but the later symptoms of vaginal bleeding can be confused with the irregular bleeding which can occur around and before the menopause. The diagnosis is made by examining the cells which can be aspirated from the cavity of the uterus as already described. In this way cells can be differentiated which have proliferated as a result of overstimulation, that is to say they are hyperplastic, and hyperplasia is suspect as a possible precancerous condition.

Various stages of hyperplasia are recognized, from Cystic Glandular Hyperplasia (CGH) to Atypical Hyperplasia (AH). These conditions may arise spontaneously from the stimulus of the body or endogenous oestrogen, or from exogenous oestrogen given as medication, although they do not, of course, necessarily progress beyond the innocent stage.

Even in experienced hands the interpretation of the microscopical findings can be very difficult. There have been suggestions, in some cases supported by photomicrographs, of misdiagnosis in the American studies. In cases of doubt, moreover, it is alleged that the bias has been towards diagnosing malignancy, and a woman's uterus removed subsequently has been found at surgery not to be cancerous after all. It has also seemed only natural in a country where, as in the USA, the rate of litigation is high, a pathologist would tend to err towards a diagnosis of malignancy than towards a benign or intermediate state, in order to be on the safe side. We know that simple hyperplasia usually reverts to normal endometrium on a progestogen. It may well be that some hyperplasia was not treated in this way, but labelled 'premalignant' or even 'malignant' The rise in endometrial cancer in the USA was possibly to some extent apparent, rather than real. This might explain the reported two-fold rise in endometrial cancer recorded between the national cancer surveys of 1948/49 and 1969/71. In spite of the rise between these years *in incidence*, the *death rate* from endometrial cancer was more than halved. If these notified cases *were* malignant a surprisingly large number got better. The incidence and death rate of breast cancer showed no rise during the same years.

Many of the instances of reported endometrial cancer arose in the sixties when around 50% of menopausal women in America were taking oestrogen, with or without supervision, in all sorts of doses, as oestrone or as oestradiol, and for all sorts of reasons, often cosmetic: the trade flourished. We shall never know the true state of the oestrogen bonanza before 1975 when the first warnings were given publicity.

## British experience

Since then prospective studies have been set up in Britain, by the Royal College of General Practitioners, the Medical Research Council, and the Committee on the Safety of Medicines, with the cooperation of numerous women in menopause clinics and their gynaecologists. Evidence is mounting of ways in which treatment can be carefully monitored to make it safe. Forewarned is to be forearmed. We know for instance that 1% of women who have spontaneously arising hyperplasia develop endometrial cancer even without taking oestrogen, that 12% with AH and 45% with severe AH do so. But where hyperplasia develops after taking oestrogen, the result is affected by the size of the dose. At King's College Hospital and the Chelsea Hospital for Women in London, Professor Stuart Campbell and Dr Malcolm Whitehead found hyperplasia developed in 33% of women on higher normal-dose regimes, but in only 18% of women on lower doses. When they added a progestogen only 5% of women on the higher doses developed hyperplasia, and none on the lower doses. In cases of spontaneously arising hyperplasia a progestogen restored the condition to normal endometrium.

Analysing the results of oestrogen treatment in over 500 women, John Studd found that 29 developed CGH and 5, AH. When they were given a progestogen the endometrium of all but one of the former and two of the latter became normal.

As more facts such as these come to light and more regular examination is carried out during combined or sequential treatment, the chances of picking up early changes will be increased, enabling avoiding action to be taken. It is important to collect information as swiftly as possible in order to balance the risk against the undoubted benefit which oestrogen can confer.

I know, for instance, one eminent American woman doctor who seven years ago had her breast removed for cancer. One year ago, on the advice of her gynaecologist, she had her uterus removed. For twenty years, in the high-dose days, she had taken oestrogen. 'I could never have held down my responsible post all those years without oestrogen' is what she says now at the age of over 60. She is well now, but had she taken a progestogen she might have been spared some anxiety, and probably surgery.

## Breast cancer

There has been some suggestion in the past that oestrogen might protect against cancer of the breast, but this conflicts with recent evidence which suggests that it may do the reverse. It was originally thought to be significant that cancer of the breast occurs more frequently in women when their oestrogen stores are low or on the decline. It is infrequent during pregnancy when the body is making a lot of oestrogen, and it is less likely to arise in women who have experienced many pregnancies, and so have been exposed to larger amounts of oestrogen than childless women; its frequency increases with age when the body's oestrogen is tailing off. It is theoretically possible that oestrogen, if given during the stage before breast cancer becomes apparent, could accelerate its development, but there has been no consistent upward trend in the death rates from breast cancer in America since the use of oestrogen has been extended. Nor has there been a rise in British figures, although it is early for any change to be noticed.

But some conditions, such as fibroadenosis of the breast, which are considered to be benign may be precancerous and there is a risk that they may progress to malignancy in women who are predisposed to breast cancer. Many surgeons and gynaecologists now consider that some other benign breast conditions preclude taking oestrogen.

An early suggestion in 1974 came from Nashville, Tennessee, that more cases of breast cancer were turning up in women who had been taking oestrogen, though the death rate had not increased correspondingly. In 1976 rather more convincing figures were given by a group of doctors in Kentucky, who had found more breast cancers than they would have expected in two thousand women who had taken oestrogen, and they thought this was of 'borderline' significance. Low doses of oestrogen had usually been given, the risk of developing breast cancer appeared to be greater the larger the dose and the longer the women were followed up. Although the risk did not appear to progress after ten years, by fifteen years it had doubled. The women who had benign breast disease were more likely to develop breast cancer, but the women at greatest risk were those who developed benign breast disease *after* they had started taking oestrogen. The investigators were concerned to find that the protection against breast cancer which usually accompanies removal of the ovaries ceased to operate after ten years. Perhaps both benign and malignant disease of the breast are influenced by oestrogen in women who are predisposed to breast disease. More research is needed here too, especially in relation to the value of progestogens. We know progesterone blocks the entry of oestrogen into the endometrial cell nucleus. It may well exert the same effect in breast tissue. If this theory is valid it could be important for a woman who has had a hysterectomy and is taking oestrogen to take a progestogen as well, even though without a uterus she could not develop endometrical cancer. *The breasts may need protection too.* It should be remembered that cancer of the breast is unfortunately a relatively common condition. There is so far no firm evidence that hormones have increased its incidence, but oestrogens might accelerate a growth.

# 11 Oestrogen the blunderbuss

The strangest aspect of the climacteric is its unpredictability in almost every respect. Why do the symptoms resulting from the lack of one particular hormone knock out some women as if by fate and leave other women untouched? Why, come to that, do menopausal symptoms ever go away? Or come in the first place?

The terminology 'Hormone Replacement Therapy' or HRT is a misnomer which is losing favour as we realize that in giving oestrogen for menopausal symptoms we are not simply replacing a commodity in short supply. We are usually over-filling an empty shelf. The doses needed to make good the deficiency more than cover the deficit, except for the small minority of women, about 10%, whose troubles are localized to the vagina and neighbouring parts. For the 75% of women whose main symptom is the hot flush the blood levels of oestrogen reached during treatment are often greatly in excess of, maybe five or more times, the levels of oestrogen in the blood which kept the individual in equilibrium before the menopause. The severity of flushing is not even related to the amount of oestrogen circulating in the body. And why do not symptoms recur every time the exogenous oestrogen is withdrawn, but only sometimes, and in some women?

Why should women who had their first period later in life, who were never married, who have never been pregnant, or who had a child when over the age of 40, or who belong to the upper socio-economic groups, come off best at the climacteric?

How is it that, except in vaginal atrophy, a placebo sometimes works as well in relieving symptoms, especially the hot flush, although we know that the latter is associated with withdrawal of the stocks of oestrogen? Why should a placebo exert such a powerful effect?

In 1977 the Boston Collaborative Drug Surveillance Programme workers published in *The Lancet* an interesting fact discovered during two surveys involving 57,000 women from twenty-four hospitals in seven different countries. Heavy smokers, they found, usually have an earlier menopause than light smokers, and light smokers tend to have an earlier menopause than women who do not smoke at all. How could smoking affect the function of the smoker's ovaries? Well, not directly. It does it through that most efficient computer of all, the brain. Nicotine probably affects the nervous centres in the brain which control the enzymes which break down the relevant hormones. Menopausal symptoms are not 'all in the mind', but they *are* all in the brain. We suspect, moreover, that some brain cells can selectively take up oestrogen into their nucleus as if by affinity. If we knew more about brain function we should be able to treat menopausal conditions with a more subtle agent than the blunderbuss oestrogen.

Meanwhile, crude as it is, we must use oestrogen for its undoubted benefits, to the best of our ability. Were I, however, in the shoes of women such as the woman doctor I described in the previous chapter, I would *in the light of our present knowledge* adhere to five rules:

1 Take oestrogen only if you really need it, to relieve distress or acute discomfort.
2 Take it in the smallest doses which will relieve symptoms: do not increase the dose without advice.
3 Take it for the shortest time necessary to prevent return of symptoms when ceasing to take it.
4 Take it sequentially, or in combination with a progestogen, especially if a bigger dose is needed, as medically advised, or if long-term treatment is necessary.
5 Take it under regular and careful supervision which will ensure that the benefits are maximized and the side effects minimized.

Not very difficult, are they, as rules go? People with common sense usually keep good rules, and these are based on common sense and born of experience. If you have got this far in this book you know now how and why these guidelines were evolved. If *you* are one of those to whom they could apply, they could completely change your attitude to the discomforts of the menopausal years and bring new and constructive hope for the next third of your life which lies ahead.

# Glossary

**adenocarcinoma** Malignancy of glandular structure.

**adenomatous hyperplasia** Overgrowth of glandular element in the lining of the uterus: cystic glandular hyperplasia synonymous.

**adrenal glands** Suprarenal glands which lie on top of each kidney and make cortisone and other hormones.

**androgen** Male sex hormone, not specific.

**androstenedione** Sex hormone with male characters. May be converted to oestrogen in the body.

**angina** Severe constricting pain, usually associated with heart conditions.

**anus** The opening of the bowel to the exterior.

**atheroma** Fatty degeneration of the inner lining of arteries, producing a yellow swelling on the internal surface.

**atherosclerosis** Arteriosclerosis, characterized by deposits of atheroma irregularly distributed in large- and medium-sized arteries and associated with fibrosis and calcification. May lead to narrowing of artery and predispose to thrombosis, angina and myocardial infarction.

**atrophy** Wasting, thinning (of tissues or organs).

**atrophic vaginitis** Thinning and atrophy of inner lining of vagina.

**calcium** Lime. Calcium salts are present in bone. Essential to life.

**calcification** Deposition of calcium salts.

**calcified** End result of calcification.

**capillaries** Minute vessels forming an intermediate system between arteries and veins.

**cerebral embolism** Embolus which lodges in the brain. One type of stroke.

**cerebral thrombosis** Clotting in a blood vessel in the brain. Also a stroke.

**cervix** The neck of the uterus, the cylindrical part between the internal and external opening.

**cholecystitis** Inflammation of the gall bladder.

**cholesterol** A fatty component. The most abundant steroid in human tissues, especially in bile and gall stones.

**climacteric** Any critical stage in human life. The period before and after the cessation of the periods, or menopause.

**clitoris** The female counterpart of the male penis. Lies between the labia minora on the vulva.

**conjugate oestrogens** Combination of an oestrogen with another substance or carrier, either natural or made chemically.

**coronary artery** Artery which supplies the heart muscle with blood.

**coronary thrombosis** Formation of clot in a coronary artery.

**corpus luteum** The structure formed in the ovary after rupture of an ovarian follicle. Makes the hormone progesterone.

**corpus uteri** The body of the uterus. Comprises two-thirds of the organ.

**curette** Instrument for scraping tissue; hence curettage, a scrape.

**cystic glandular hyperplasia** Overgrowth of the glands which are present in the endometrium with the formation of cysts.

**cystitis** Inflammation of the urinary bladder.

**dienoestrol** A synthetic oestrogen.

**dydrogesterone** The progestogen which does not prevent ovulation.

**dyspareunia** Painful sexual intercourse, usually related to the female.

**embolus** Any foreign substance such as a detached part of a clot circulating in the blood and forming an obstruction at the place of its lodgement.

**embryo** The stage of development within the uterus from conception until approximately the end of the second month.

**embryology** Science of the origin and development of the embryo. Adjective: embryological.

**endogenous** Originating or produced within the body.

**endometriosis** Condition in which endometrial tissue arises in abnormal situation outside the uterus, commonly the ovary, wall of uterus or other organs. Contains blood.

**endometrium** The mucous membrane which lines the uterus. It contains simple glands like tubes, which open on to the inner surface.

**enzyme** A protein made by body cells which acts as a catalyst and induces changes in other substances while remaining unchanged itself.

**ethinyloestradiol** A synthetic oestrogen.

**exogenous** Originating or produced outside the body.

**fallopian tube** Structure attached to the uterus through which the ovum passes from the ovary.

**fibrin** A protein-containing substance formed during clotting of blood.

**fibroid** Benign tumour of the uterus, consists of muscle and fibrous

144

material. Mainly arises during reproductive period of life, usually regresses after menopause.

**follicle (ovarian)** A small sac in the ovary containing an egg.

**formication** Sensation of ants creeping over the skin. 'Pins and needles'.

**gall bladder** A sac under the liver. Stores bile and passes it down the bile duct to the intestine.

**gall stones** Stones, usually composed of cholesterol crystals, in gall bladder or bile duct.

**glycogen** 'Animal starch'. A carbohydrate present in nearly all body tissues, the principal carbohydrate reserve, readily converted to glucose.

**gonad** Sexual gland, testicle or ovary. Adjective: gonadal.

**gonadotrophins** Hormones of pituitary origin which promote growth and function of gonads in both sexes.

**hexoestrol** A synthetic oestrogen.

**hormone** A chemical substance made by the ductless glands, which brings about specific changes via the bloodstream in distant cells and organs.

**hydroxyproline** An amino acid which produces natural sugar.

**hyperlipidaemia** Abnormally high proportion of fats in blood.

**hyperplasia** Increase in cells. Overgrowth.

**hypothalamus** Area of mid-brain which controls independent functions including the emotions.

**infarct** Death of tissue due to withdrawal of blood supply.

**infarction** Development of an infarct.

**labia (majora and minora)** Part of the external female genitalia. Narrow lip-shaped folds which bind the front part of the opening of the vagina and cover the clitoris.

**lactation** Production of breast milk.

**libido** Sexual desire.

**lipids** Fats.

**lipidaemia** Presence of fats in blood.

**lipoproteins** Complex compounds containing fat and protein.

**menarche** The first menstruation. Establishment of menstrual function.

**menopause** Final cessation of menstruation. The last period.

**mestranol** Ethinyloestradiol-3-methyl ether. Synthetic oestrogen with similar action to oestradiol.

**myocardium** The muscular wall of the heart.

**norethisterone** A progestogen.

**norgestrel** A progestogen.

**oestradiol** A free natural oestrogen.

**oestriol** A free natural oestrogen.

**oestrogen** Female sex hormone.

**oestrone** A free natural oestrogen.

**osteoporosis** Loss of bony tissue due to lack of calcium. Skeletal atrophy. Porous condition of bone.

**ovary** Female sex gland.

**ovulation** Escape of egg (ovum) from ovarian follicle.

**parathyroid gland** One of four ductless or endocrine glands. Lies adjacent to thyroid gland. Produces parathyroid hormone.

**pelvis** Bony hip girdle.

**perineum** The area between the thighs from the vulva to the anus. Adjective: perineal.

**phosphate** Salt of phosphoric acid.

**phosphorus** Non-metallic element.

**pituitary gland** Ductless gland at base of brain. Makes pituitary hormones, gonadotrophins and others.

**placenta** Structure formed in pregnancy on the inner wall of the uterus to nourish the foetus. Is attached to the umbilical cord. Makes oestrogen.

**platelets** Microscopic blood structures associated with clot formation.

**precursor** An inactive substance that is converted to an active enzyme vitamin, hormone or chemical substance. Anything from which another is derived.

**progesterone** The hormone of the corpus luteum of the ovary. Induces endometrial change after ovulation and the early changes in pregnancy.

**progestogen** A synthetic substance possessing the same pharmacological properties as progesterone.

**prolapse** Dropping or protrusion. Usually applied to rectum or vagina.

**proliferation** Formation of new tissue or multiplication of cells. In the uterine lining occurs in the first half of the menstrual cycle.

**proliferative hyperplasia** Overgrowth (of endometrium).

**pruritus** Extreme itching, usually referred to anus or vulva.

**psychometric testing** The measurement of the duration and force of mental processes.

**puberty** The growth and development of the secondary sexual characteristics. The onset of the reproductive period of life.

**pulmonary embolism** An embolus which lodges in the lung.

**rectum** Lower segment of bowel.

**sperm** Semen; produced by testes.

**sphincter** Muscular ring which closes an orifice.

**steroids** A large family of chemical substances comprising many hormones, body constituents including oestrogens and testosterone, drugs, each built upon a typical 4-ring nucleus.

**stilboestrol** A synthetic oestrogen.

**surgical menopause** An artificial menopause produced by removal of ovaries.

**testis (es plural)** Male reproductive gland(s).

**testosterone** The most potent naturally occurring androgen. Formed in testes, and adrenals and in the ovary (from the precursor androstenedione).

**thrombus** A clot formed during life in a blood vessel.

**thrombo-embolism** Embolism from detachment of clot.

**thrombosis** Clotting.

**triglyceride** Combination of glycerol and a fatty acid. Most animal and vegetable fats are triglyceride esters.

**urethra** Channel through which urine is excreted, extends from bladder to surface of the perineum.

**uterus** Womb.

**vagina** The genital canal from the uterus to the vulva.

**vaginitis** Inflammation of the vagina.

**vasomotor** Causing dilatation or constriction of blood vessels, regulating the tension in blood vessels.

**virilization** The development of masculine characteristics.

**vulva** Female external genitalia.

# List of menopause clinics: NHS and private

**London: NHS**
**Menopause clinics at the following hospitals:**

Chelsea Hospital for Women, Dept of Obstetrics & Gynaecology,
Dovehouse Street,
London SW3 6LT (01 352 6446)
Dulwich Hospital, East Dulwich Grove, Dulwich,
London SE22 3PT (01 693 3377)
The Hospital for Women ('Soho Hospital') (part of Middlesex
Hospital group), Soho Square,
London W1 V6JB (01 580 7928)
King's College Hospital, Dept of Obstetrics & Gynaecology,
Denmark Hill,
London SE5 9RS (01 274 6222)
Royal Free Hospital, Pond Street,
London NW3 2Q9 (01 794 0500)
St Thomas' Hospital, Dept of Gynaecology, Lambeth Palace Road,
London SE1 7EH (01 928 9292)
Samaritan Hospital for Women, Marylebone Road,
London NW1 5YE (01 402 4211)

*also*:

Family Centre, Wood Street, Barnet, Herts


**London; private**

The Menopause Clinic, 148 Harley Street,
London W1 (01 935 1900)
The Menopause Clinic, 56 Harley Street,
London W1 N1AE (01 580 1143)
The Menopause Clinic, 56 Anerley Park,
London SE20 8NB (01 778 8027)
The Nuffield Centre (BUPA), Webb House, 210 Pentonville Road,
London W1 9TA (01 278 4565/4647)
The Well Woman Centre, Marie Stopes House, 108 Whitfield Street,
London W1P 6BE (01 388 0662)

*also*:

The Menopause Clinic, 9 South Road, Twickenham,
Middlesex (01 977 6099)


## England: NHS

St Chad's Hospital, Hagley Road, Edgbaston,
BIRMINGHAM (021 454 4151)
Birmingham & Midland Hospital for Women, Showall Green Lane,
BIRMINGHAM 11 (021 722 1101)
Dudley Hospital, Dept of Obstetrics & Gynaecology,
BIRMINGHAM 18 (021 554 3801)
Women's Hospital, Professorial Unit, Queen Elizabeth Medical
Centre, Edgbaston,
BIRMINGHAM B15 2TG (Harborne 021 472 1377)
Royal Sussex Hospital, Dept of Obstetrics & Gynaecology,
BRIGHTON, Sussex (0273 66611)
The Lady Chichester Hospital, Dept of Obstetrics & Gynaecology,
New Church Street,
HOVE, Sussex (0273 778383)
South Mead Hospital, Westbury on Trim,
BRISTOL (Bristol 622321)
Dryburn Hospital, Dept of Obstetrics & Gynaecology,
DURHAM (Durham 64911)
Women's Hospital, Dept of Obstetrics & Gynaecology,
LEEDS (453905)
The General Infirmary, MRC Mineral Metabolism Unit,
LEEDS (32759)
Women's Hospital, Gynaecological Clinic, Catherine Street,
LIVERPOOL (051 709 5461)
LONDON (see separate list page 149)
Manchester General Hospital, Crumpsall,
MANCHESTER M8 6RB (061 740 1444)
Wythenshaw Hospital, MANCHESTER 22
(061 998 7070) (Wednesdays)
City Hospital, Dept of Obstetrics & Gynaecology, Hucknall Road,
NOTTINGHAM (608111)
George Eliot Hospital, Dept of Obstetrics & Gynaecology,
College Street,
NUNEATON (4201)

The John Radcliffe Hospital, Dept of Obstetrics & Gynaecology,
OXFORD (64711)
Peterborough & District Hospital, Thorpe Road,
PETERBOROUGH, Northants (0733 67451)
Jessop Hospital, University Department,
SHEFFIELD (25291)
Stafford General Infirmary, Dept of Obstetrics & Gynaecology,
STAFFORD (0785 58251)
Ashford Hospital,
STAINES, Middlesex (07842 51188)
Stepping Hill Hospital, Dept of Obstetrics & Gynaecology,
STOCKPORT, Cheshire (061 483 1010)

## England: private

The Menopause Clinic, 10-12 Leahurst Crescent, Harbone,
BIRMINGHAM B17 0LG (021 427 6525)
The Menopause Clinic, 48 Whitegate Drive,
BLACKPOOL (0253 32647)
The Richmond Hill Clinic, 21 Richmond Hill, Clifton,
BRISTOL BS8 1BA (0272 36084)
Menopause Clinic, 31 Rodney Street,
LIVERPOOL L1 9EH (051 709 8522)
**London (see separate list page 149)**
Menopause Clinic, 16 St John Street,
MANCHESTER 1 (061 834 3133)
Wavertree Clinic, 6 Bradwell Lane,
NEWCASTLE, Staffs (561218)
Nuffield Clinic, Osborne Road,
NEWCASTLE UPON TYNE (0632 815331)
The Health Centre, Churchtown,
SOUTHPORT, Lancs (24411)

## Northern Ireland: NHS

Samaritan Hospital, (Dr J. F. O'Sullivan), Lisburn Road,
BELFAST (41316)

## Eire

Coombe Hospital, (Dr Niall Duignan),
DUBLIN 8 (0001 757561)

## Scotland: NHS

Aberdeen University, Gynaecology & Endocrine Clinic, Foresthill,
ABERDEEN (23423)
Royal Infirmary, Gynaecological Outpatients, Dept of Obstetrics
& Gynaecology, 39 Chalmers Street,
EDINBURGH EH3 9ER (Newington) 031 667 1011
Glasgow Royal Infirmary, Gynaecological Clinic, Castle Street,
GLASGOW G4 0NA (Bell) 041 552 3535
Redlands Hospital for Women, Lancaster Crescent,
GLASGOW (041 339 2226)
Western Infirmary & Stophill General Hospital,
GLASGOW (041 339 8822)

## Scotland: private

Royal Scottish Nursing Home, Menopause Clinic,
19 Drumsheugh Gardens,
EDINBURGH 3 (031 225 3881)
The Bellgrove Clinic, 556 Gallowgate,
GLASGOW G40 2PA  (041 554 7157)

## Wales: NHS

St Tydfil's Hospital, Dept of Obstetrics & Gynaecology,
MERTHYR TYDFIL (3401)

## Wales: the clinic below is NOT NHS, but FREE to patients

Simbech Research Centre, The Menopause Clinic,
MERTHYR TYDFIL (2324)

*also*:

A clinic expected to open in CARDIFF soon.

# Index

# Dr David Delvin
## for the Back Pain Association
# You and Your Back 60p

However young and fit you are, it's more than likely that you will one day suffer back trouble.

Back pain is unpleasant and a nuisance. It costs the country £300,000,000 a year in medical care, sickness benefit and lost production. The cost in suffering and disability is incalculable.

Dr Delvin explains how your back should function; what sort of back trouble you could suffer; how to cope with back trouble and how to prevent it happening to you.

# Diana Davenport
# One-Parent Families 85p

More than a million people in Britain have to be Mum and Dad at the same time. If you're one of them, this handbook is designed specifically for you. Diana Davenport, a working journalist with a wealth of first-hand experience of running a one-parent family, tackles the enormous range of problems faced by a parent without a marriage partner – housing, legal problems, the psychological and logistic headaches of jobs, school holidays, babysitters.

# Mariane Kohler
# The Secrets of Relaxation £1

True relaxation is the key to the release of mental and physical strain. As well as the lesser known exotic approaches to relaxation, Miss Kohler presents the age-old methods of yoga and meditation that pave the way to the individual's mastery over his emotions and bring both bodily health and inner peace.

## Dr Richard Mackarness
## **Not All In The Mind** 70p

In this new vitally important book, Dr Richard Mackarness, doctor and psychiatrist, shows how millions may be made ill, physically and mentally, by common foods such as milk, eggs, coffee and white flour.

He relates case after case from his clinical practice where patients with chronic ailments resistant to other methods of treatment were cured by identifying and eliminating foods to which they had developed unsuspected allergy.

## Dr E. K. Lederman
## **Good Health through Natural Therapy** 75p

Convenience foods, lack of exercise, stress, smoking and drinking are all to blame for the 'diseases of affluence'. With this book – written by a highly qualified Harley Street specialist – you can raise your own health standards: the right diet, the right exercise and proper relaxation. You will learn how the natural healing of the homeopath and osteopath can be of real help to everyone.

## Dr Andrew Stanway
## **Taking the Rough with the Smooth** 70p

The discovery that foods rich in dietary fibre (roughage) can help prevent the serious diseases of the affluent society has been heralded as the medical breakthrough of the decade. This is the definitive book on the subject written for the general reader.

Mouthwatering high-fibre recipes are included to enable readers to adapt their diets for a happier and healthier life.

D. C. Jarvis
## Folk Medicine 75p

The tough, hard-living mountain folk of the state of Vermont have a time-honoured folk medicine.

The late Dr Jarvis, a fifth generation native of Vermont, lived and practised among these sturdy people for over fifty years. This book is the result of his deep study of their way of life and in particular of their concepts of diet. These he was able to test against his formal medical training and prove by long experience.

He offers a new theory on the treatment and prevention of a wide variety of ailments – the common cold, hay fever, arthritis, high blood pressure, chronic fatigue, overweight and many others – and holds out a promise of zestful good health for young and old.

## Arthritis and Folk Medicine 70p

When folk medicine swept through Britain and America with its amazing message of relief from countless diseases, the author received innumerable letters from sufferers from arthritis, lumbago, gout and muscular rheumatism, enquiring what Folk Medicine had to offer them for their misery.

Now Dr Jarvis replies – explaining step by step a simple, sensible method of treatment, evolved through generations of trial and error by the rugged folk of his native Vermont and meticulously tested against his own medical experience.